Hoʻi Hou Ka Mauli Ola

Published by University of Hawai'i Press
in Association with

Hawai'inuiākea School of Hawaiian Knowledge
University of Hawai'i at Mānoa
Dean Maenette K. P. Ah Nee-Benham

Hawai'inuiākea is available online through
Project MUSE (http://muse.jhu.edu).

Hawai'inuiākea No. 5

Ho'i Hou Ka Mauli Ola
Pathways to Native Hawaiian Health

Edited by
Winona K. Mesiona Lee and Mele A. Look

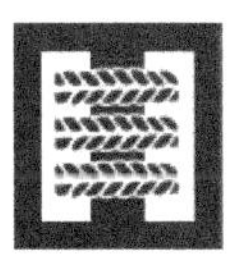

Hawai'inuiākea School of Hawaiian Knowledge

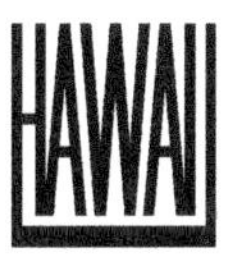

University of Hawai'i Press

Honolulu

Printed in the United States of America

22 21 20 19 18 6 5 4 3 2

Library of Congress Cataloging-in-Publication Data

Names: Lee, Winona K. Mesiona, editor | Look, Mele A., editor | Blaisdell, Richard K. (Richard Kekuni), dedicatee.
Title: Ho'i hou ka mauli ola = Pathways to native Hawaiian health / edited by Winona K. Mesiona Lee and Mele A. Look.
Other titles: Pathways to native Hawaiian health | Hawai'inuiākea monograph; 5.
Description: Honolulu : University of Hawai'i Press in association with Hawai'inuiākea School of Hawaiian Knowledge, [2017] | Series: Hawai'inuiākea ; no. 5 | Dedicated to Richard Kekuni Akana Blaisdell (1925-2016). | Includes bibliographical references.
Identifiers: LCCN 2017005474 | ISBN 9780824872731 (pbk. ; alk. paper)
Subjects: LCSH: Hawaiians—Health and hygiene. | Medical care—Hawaii. | Hawaiians—Medicine. | Medicine—Study and teaching (Graduate)—Hawaii.
Classification: LCC RA448.5.H38 H65 2017 | DDC 362.1089/9942—dc23
LC record available at https://lccn.loc.gov/2017005474

Cover image:
Ola Nā Iwi, by Puni Jackson, acrylic on canvas, 78″ x 66″, 2010.
A self-portrait, the image depicts a moment of clarity and prayer atop Haleakalā. Through oli and in our sacred wahi pana, we open ourselves to the connection between Papa and Wākea, earth and sky, past and present, kūpuna and mo'opuna. We become the space between, where the bones of our ancestors continue to live even in the vibration of our voices. Aloha 'āina, ola nā kūpuna!

University of Hawai'i Press books are printed on acid-free paper and meet the guidelines for permanence and durability of the Council on Library Resources.

This volume is dedicated to Richard Kekuni Akana Blaisdell (1925–2016), who encouraged generations to be compassionate healers, courageous scientists, resilient activists, and invigorated teachers. Ho'oulu lāhui!

Contents

From the Dean

Welina mai kākou!

Mahalo nui loa for picking up the fifth volume in the *Hawai'inuiākea* series, which publishes high-quality research and inquiry, kūpuna reflections, and artistic expressions. The series aims to advance Kanaka Maoli perspectives, *'ike* that seamlessly integrates knowledge and discoveries at the intersection of socio-political, cultural-historical, economic and ecological science, and indigenous knowing. The series' scope is truly transdisciplinary as it seeks to speak to new ideas within the context of ancient knowledge and contemporary conundrums; to engage the diversity of our Kanaka scholars from the social sciences to the humanities, to ecology, to art, to health and well-being, to law, to language and linguistics, and so forth. It is our hope to connect methodologies and practices that are innovative and that ensure clear practices and policies for the betterment of our lāhui.

We all have much to learn from the holistic perspectives, practices, and expertise derived from centuries of knowledge that link our health and well-being with our ecosystems. One might begin this study with the challenges this presents to a Western scientific community. This volume, however, asks the reader to begin at a very different starting point, that is, at the intersections of the spiritual, ancestral, cultural, and environmental factors of health and well-being.

The 'ōlelo no'eau, *'a'ohe pau ka 'ike i ka hālau ho'okahi,*[1] speaks to the concept of the sacredness of relations. At the core of one's life is the truth that every individual is related to the people in one's immediate family and social group, as well as to the physical environment and spiritual world. It is through these relations that we build strong *'auwai* for Kānaka Maoli to be advocates for their health and well-being.

So at the heart of this framing is the imperative that health research and methodologies begin with an indigenous perspective—in this case, *'ike kanaka 'ōiwi*—as it evolves and finds synergies with other indigenous and non-indigenous knowledge systems. The authors and contributors to this volume, members or partners with the Department of Native Hawaiian Health in the John A. Burns School of Medicine at the University of Hawai'i at Mānoa, are building foundations and approaches to Native Hawaiian well-being that fully consider traditional expertise in culturally appropriate health research and practice. Each contribution is strengthened by the collective impact of the whole as it tangles with the web of contexts within which the authors work to ensure the health and well-being of all Hawai'i's people.

Na'u me ka ha'aha'a!
Dr. Maenette K. P. Ah Nee-Benham, Dean
Hawai'inuiākea School of Hawaiian Knowledge
University of Hawai'i at Mānoa

NOTE

1. M. K. Pukui, *'Ōlelo No'eau: Hawaiian Proverbs and Poetical Sayings* (Honolulu: Bishop Museum Press, 1983), 24.

Editors' Note

Mauli means life, heart, seat of life, spirit, and even ghost. It is our essential nature, our very being. *Ola* means well-being, healthy. To bring back the state of vibrant health for Native Hawaiians is our singular objective, the pathway we travel, the passion of our authors, and the focus of this book. The title of this volume is a phrase found in traditional chants calling forth life, and is in fact from the *pule ho'ōla* written for the *māla lā'au lapa'au,* the Hawaiian medicinal garden at the University of Hawai'i medical school.

The contributions that form this book come from thirty-three authors, nearly all of whom are part of the newest department at the John A. Burns School of Medicine at the University of Hawai'i at Mānoa (JABSOM). The Department of Native Hawaiian Health (DNHH) serves as a unique resource, being the only clinical department in a U.S. medical school dedicated to the health of an indigenous population. The authors are representative of the many disciplines, strategies, and projects working to find solutions to health problems, cures to diseases, improvements to health care for Hawaiians and Pacific Islanders, and pathways to grow new doctors and researchers.

Dr. Keawe Kaholokula, respected scientist, clinician, and chair of the DNNH, sets an excellent foundation for the chapters that follow by providing a historical perspective on Hawaiian health and proposing futures based on demographics and social movements. Dr. Kaholokula represents a growing cadre of Hawaiian scientists who work to uncover new knowledge by applying excellence in medical and research training fastened securely to a foundation of traditional Hawaiian knowledge. Increasingly, these individuals are fluent speakers of the Hawaiian language and are skilled cultural practitioners, providing them the invaluable capacity to access a vast repository of written and oral Hawaiian scholarship that includes original, first-person accounts of viewpoints and practices on healing, health, and well-being.

Perhaps most significantly, the community projects, medical research, quantitative findings, and educational programs described in this volume are built on the contributions of those who came before, and on whose shoulders we stand. Thus, it is with profound regard and great pleasure that we dedicate this book to a beloved kupuna, Dr. Richard Kekuni Blaisdell, one of the founding faculty members of JABSOM and a mentor to several generations of healers, activists, educators, and scientists. He is an essential voice in any conversation about Hawaiian health. Indeed, each of the chapters was a subject of great interest to him. And it is a singular distinction to have an archival interview with Kekuni included in this book. Also distinctive to this volume is an insightful chapter about research and cultural practice by renowned kumu hula Māpuana de Silva, and an *oli komo,* a welcoming chant, written by Dr. Marcus Iwane, a young Hawaiian physician.

Various authors share their personal journeys to becoming doctors and highlight the contributions of pioneers Drs. Benjamin Young and Nanette Judd, who worked tirelessly to advocate and support Native Hawaiian students' dreams of becoming physicians. Also included is a history of the Hansen's disease settlement at Kalaupapa as well as the efforts of a nationally recognized biomedical researcher and epigeneticist, Alika Maunakea, to develop more Hawaiian scientists. Each author endeavored to write to a broad audience to make the collective work accessible to as many readers as possible, and as editors, *we* endeavored to limit the occurrence of medical jargon, much to the chagrin of the authors, most of whom are doctors and scientists!

Our goal with this publication is to illuminate the vast, varied, and fascinating work that doctors, researchers, and healthcare providers engage in to improve the health of Native Hawaiians and Pacific Islanders. The relevance of their work impacts all of us regardless of ethnicity: the discoveries made in the search for solutions to health problems apply not only to other indigenous communities, but to all who call Hawai'i home.

Ki'eki'e Lanihuli

Marcus Kawika Iwane and 'Ānela K. Nacapoy Iwane

Ki'eki'e Lanihuli,
Linohau i ka ulu lehua
Ua noe o Konahuanui,
Ka 'iu kau i ka hano
Hanohano Waipuhia,
Ka wai ho'oma'ū i ke oho palai
I laila 'o Māmala
Lamalama i ka lei pāpahi
Hia'ai ke 'ike aku
He leo kāhea e komo mai ē

Lanihuli stands majestically
Beautifully decorated in groves of lehua
Konahuanui is enveloped with cold mists
Its peak placed in the highest honor
Well known is Waipuhia
The "upside-down" waterfall that moistens and cools the ferns
Māmala is in plain view
Vivacious and glowing with adornments
Very pleasing to the eye
Heed the call, a call to enter

Mauli Ola:
Pathways to Optimal Kanaka ʻŌiwi Health

Joseph Keaweʻaimoku Kaholokula

Centuries before the arrival of European settlers to Hawaiʻi, our Kanaka ʻŌiwi (Native Hawaiian) ancestors developed an elaborate and highly sophisticated public health system based on the concepts of *kapu* (people, places, and things held under strict regulation) and *noa* (people, places, and things free of restriction).[1] Referred to as the Kapu system, it was essentially a public health system based on socio-religious tenets to ensure equitable access to natural resources and the availability of these resources in perpetuity.[2] These resources were strictly controlled, such as the use of fresh water and fishing. As part of this resource management effort, there was a division of labor by social ranking, which ascribed different sets of behaviors and privileges to each. By all accounts, it was a highly effective public health system that ensured the availability and distribution of life-sustaining resources that minimized if not eliminated starvation, disease, and illness on islands with finite resources.

The observations of Captain James Cook and his men in 1778 suggest the effectiveness of the Kapu system and the health status of our ancestors. They noted that the natives were "...above middle size, strong, well made...a fine handsome set of people," and that they were "truly good natured, social, friendly, and humane, possessing much liveliness and...good humour."[3] Surely, these descriptors are indicative of a healthy and thriving native population at the dawn of permanent contact with Westerners.[4]

Although it has been criticized as being an oppressive socio-religious order, favoring the elite in ancient society, the Kapu system was based on similar principles and enforceable regulations to the modern public health systems in most developed countries today. For example, fresh water is still one of the most precious natural resources, required for drinking, cooking, and farming, which is still regulated by government. How resources are allocated, distributed, and accessed today continues to vary considerably by social ranking. Even the distribution of labor is still based on social ranking, reflected in terms such as blue-collar versus white-collar workers and jobs.

Unlike the ancient Kapu system, however, the modern Western version, better referred to as capitalism, has resulted in large health inequities for contemporary Kānaka ʻŌiwi. Under U.S. occupation, the rates of mental and physical illnesses, such as depression and diabetes, have been considerably higher among Kānaka 'Ōiwi compared to all other major ethnic groups in Hawai'i.[5] Kānaka 'Ōiwi have also experienced greater social and economic disadvantages in education, employment, incarceration, and housing.[6] In this chapter, my perspectives on the social and cultural determinants of health for Kānaka 'Ōiwi, the opportunities I see on the horizon for improving these determinants, and our aspirations as Kānaka 'Ōiwi in achieving optimal health are explored.

My perspectives explored here are based on my experiences as a Kanaka 'Ōiwi and as a health professional working with, and on behalf of, other Kānaka 'Ōiwi. My motivation for writing this perspective piece is to move the dialogue in the health inequities field from talking about "disadvantages and risks" to talking about "advantages and opportunities." My desire with this piece is that health professionals, researchers, and policy makers will develop a stronger appreciation for the "root causes" for the disproportionate burden of physical and mental health issues among Kānaka 'Ōiwi as well as the cultural strengths already in place to advance Kanaka 'Ōiwi health. My other desire is that we, as Kānaka 'Ōiwi, take full advantage of our shared aspirations and cultural resources to advance our health and well-being. To begin my exploration, I offer a definition of health from a Kanaka 'Ōiwi perspective.

An Indigenous Perspective of Health

Mauli Ola is the "breath of life" or "power of healing."[7] It is often used to refer to a person's health as reflected in the 'ōlelo no'eau (proverb) "kihe, a Mauliola" (sneeze, and may you have life). Mauli Ola is also the deity of health embodied by the natural elements as reflected in the 'ōlelo no'eau "Ka lā i ka Mauliola" (The sun at the source of life).[8] It reflects the reciprocal person–environment relationship important to well-being; that is, optimal health is shaped by one's relationship to his or her spirituality and the natural elements.

I use the concept of Mauli Ola in this chapter to refer to health and define it here as a "balanced" state of spiritual, physical, mental, and social well-being beyond the mere absence of disease or disability.[9] These aspects of well-being are related to the quality of a person's spiritual, interpersonal, and environmental relationships as reflected in the traditional Kanaka 'Ōiwi values around ho'omana (reverence), 'ohana (filial piety), mālama 'āina (caring for the land), and aloha 'āina (land stewardship and patriotism to Hawai'i). The optimal balance amongst these areas of well-being is based on a person's subjective experience, and this optimal balance can differ across Kānaka 'Ōiwi.

Social and Cultural Determinants of Mauli Ola

Although genetic (e.g., inherited traits), biological (e.g., metabolic abnormalities), and behavioral (e.g., eating and exercise habits) determinants of Mauli Ola are often the focus of attention, the social determinants of Mauli Ola are equally important, that is, the societal, political, and economic forces that influence the social structure and hierarchy and the distribution of power, resources, and opportunities in society that differentially impact the health and well-being of people.[10] Most impacted by the adverse consequences of these social determinants are indigenous and ethnic minority populations who are overrepresented in poorer socioeconomic conditions and who also have higher morbidity and mortality rates than Caucasians.[11] A scientific review of studies published over a seven-year period concluded that there is little evidence for a clear genetic explanation of the cardiovascular disease disparities seen between Blacks and Whites in the United States.[12] It is likely that these disparities are better accounted for by environmental (e.g., obesiogenic neighborhoods) and social (e.g., discrimination) factors,[13] and that these "upstream" factors can shape the biological and behavioral determinants of health.[14]

For Indigenous Peoples living under the rule of foreign settlers, such as Kānaka 'Ōiwi, the preservation of cultural traditions (e.g., native language, values, and practices) and sacred places, access to ancestral lands, a strong indigenous identity, and cultural participation are also important, positive determinants of Mauli Ola.[15] However, these indigenous values, practices, and aspirations are often challenged by those of the settler society and other ethnic groups. A history of physical, emotional, and cultural marginalization due to discriminatory acts and compulsory acculturation strategies (e.g., banning of native language), many of which still persist today, have negatively impacted the Mauli Ola of Indigenous Peoples[16]—a phenomenon often referred to as historical or cultural trauma.[17]

Studies of Kānaka 'Ōiwi illustrate how historical trauma might be manifested in the present: the perception and experience of historical trauma among Kanaka 'Ōiwi college students are associated with more substance use (alcohol, cigarettes, and/or marijuana) for those who also report more discrimination, whereas for those with a high degree of pride in being Kānaka 'Ōiwi, it is associated with less substance use.[18] Higher levels of perceived discrimination in Kānaka 'Ōiwi are associated with a higher risk for hypertension and dysregulation in the stress hormone cortisol.[19] Cultural loss and threats to indigenous identity among Kānaka 'Ōiwi have been linked to depression.[20]

From left to right of the model depicted in Figure 2.1: Consider how population decimation, conversion to Christianity and its condemnation of tradi-

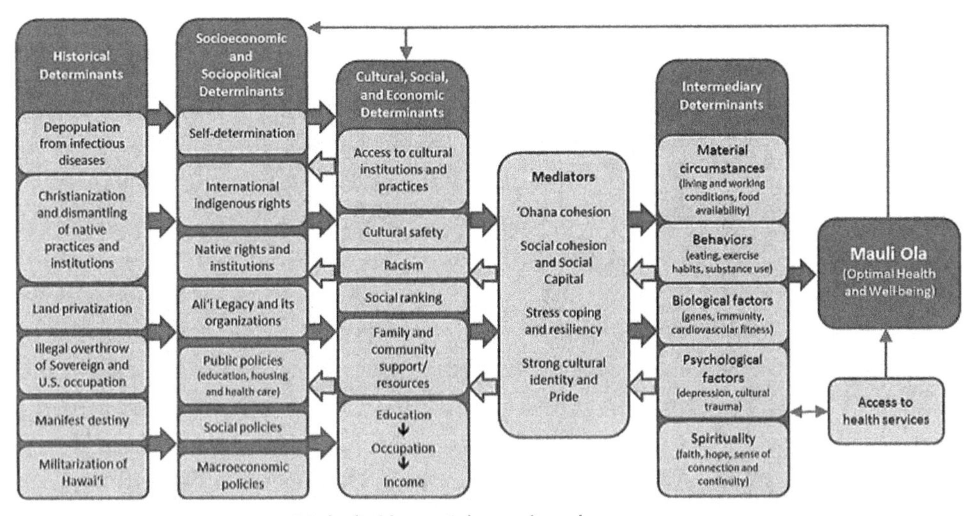

Mohala i ka wai, ka maka o ka pua

Flowers thrive where this is water, as thriving people are found where living conditions are good

Figure 2.1. Social and Cultural Determinants of Mauli Ola for Kānaka ʻŌiwi.

tional values and practices, land privatization, and loss of political control in the 1800s, and the militarization of Hawaiʻi, banning of the Hawaiian language, tourism, migrations, and foreign investments of the 1900s have led to the current state of affairs for Kānaka ʻŌiwi. Although these past events are non-modifiable, they have led to the displacement and marginalization of Kānaka ʻŌiwi in our own homeland and to disadvantages in education, housing, and workforce—factors that are modifiable. Consider how the resulting political system and its decisions, such as how resources are distributed and how public policies might favor the interest of one group over another, can impact the safety (e.g., crime and environmental toxins) and availability of resources (e.g., walking trails and usable sidewalks) in a particular neighborhood, worksite, or public school system; how the safety and available resources of these environments can impact whether or not a person has access to fresh fruits and vegetables, safe and clean parks, and the best educational opportunities; how the availability and affordability of healthy food options and physical activity venues can affect whether or not a person is obese or develops diabetes; and how access to quality health care can prevent (or bring about), delay (versus early onset), or manage a person's health problems. Finally, consider how all these factors are not equally distributed or accessible across communities and ethnic groups and how the added burden of discrimination, economic deprivation, and cultural threats can adversely impact these factors.

Despite the socioeconomic and sociocultural factors that have positioned Kānaka ʻŌiwi at a disadvantage in Hawaiʻi, the adverse health effects are tempered by the social, educational, and health care institutions of our Ali'i (Royal) Legacy and public policies. Imagine what the educational situation for Kānaka 'Ōiwi would be like if not for the existence of Kamehameha Schools, the legacy of Princess Bernice Pauahi Bishop. Imagine what the fate of many desolate and orphaned Kanaka 'Ōiwi children would have been if not for the social services provided by the Queen Lili'uokalani Children's Center. Imagine what would have become of many Kūpuna (elders) if not for the Lunalilo Home. Imagine what health care would be like for many Kānaka 'Ōiwi without the existence of The Queen's Health Systems, the legacy of Queen Emma and King Kamehameha IV. And, imagine what the conditions would be like for many Kānaka 'Ōiwi without the Office of Hawaiian Affairs (OHA) and the governmental support received through the Hawaiian Homes Commission Act, the Native Hawaiian Education Act, and the Native Hawaiian Health Care Improvement Act. No doubt, the legacy of our Ali'i, OHA, and targeted public laws have had a tremendous, positive impact on Mauli Ola for Kānaka 'Ōiwi.

Future Opportunities for Mauli Ola

I see several opportunities on the horizon for Kānaka 'Ōiwi that could expedite the improvement of our social and cultural determinants of Mauli Ola, if we can capitalize on and strategically leverage these opportunities. They are linked to 1) the projected demographic trends in the Kanaka 'Ōiwi population, 2) the continued cultural revitalization, 3) the broader participation in society, and 4) the self-determination and the international indigenous movement.

Demographic Trends

Several positive demographic changes in our Kanaka 'Ōiwi population are expected to occur over the next 30 years that could facilitate Mauli Ola. It is estimated that, by the year 2045, the Kanaka 'Ōiwi population in Hawai'i will almost double in size from its current 298,000 to 512,000.[21] Most of this increase will occur among Kānaka 'Ōiwi under 35 years of age with modest increases among those 65 and older. Kānaka 'Ōiwi are expected to continue having children at higher rates than most other ethnic groups, consistent with the value of 'ohana. Although the current life expectancy of Kānaka 'Ōiwi is a decade shorter than most other ethnic groups,[22] our life expectancy is predicted to increase, albeit this increase will likely remain less than most other ethnic groups in Hawai'i.

It is hoped that, along with the population doubling, the number of Kānaka 'Ōiwi with college qualifications will increase. Although the percentage of Kānaka 'Ōiwi enrolling in college currently appears to have reached a plateau at 14 percent versus the overall state at 30 percent,[23] there are collaborative efforts between the University of Hawai'i and Kamehameha Schools that will surely contribute to an upward trend in this area. An increase in college graduation rates will bring greater economic advancement and improvements in quality of life for many Kānaka 'Ōiwi, given that a higher education level is strongly associated with higher incomes and lower mortality and morbidity.[24]

The population recovery of Kānaka 'Ōiwi is remarkable and a sign of resiliency and vitality. Based on a new demographic analysis technique, it is estimated the Kanaka 'Ōiwi population was at 683,000 in 1778.[25] Considering that the Kanaka 'Ōiwi population declined by 95 percent (to about 30,000) in the late 1800s, mostly due to infectious diseases introduced by European settlers for which our ancestors had no natural immunity,[26] the estimated doubling of our population over the next thirty years, a rise that started in the 1940s, is a phenomenal "comeback" story. The greatest challenge now to our physical health is chronic diseases, such as diabetes and heart disease, which are linked to our higher rates of obesity, high blood pressure and cholesterol, and cigarette smoking.[27]

The demographic changes in our Kanaka 'Ōiwi population over the next 30 years can be a tremendous advantage for realizing Mauli Ola. At our current population size of 298,000, Kānaka 'Ōiwi make up nearly a quarter of Hawai'i's overall population where there is supposedly no numerically dominant ethnic group. By 2045, we are likely to make up one-third of this population with 512,000 Kānaka 'Ōiwi.[28] Imagine the political influence Kānaka 'Ōiwi could amass by making up a third of the population. Although the issue of how self-determination should be achieved or look like (e.g., through U.S. federal recognition or de-occupation by the United States) remains a source of contention amongst many Kānaka 'Ōiwi, it does not preclude us from seeking other avenues within the current political system to advance our collective Mauli Ola. Imagine the political leverage we could possess as Kānaka 'Ōiwi with the development of such a critical mass and our potential increased numbers across the academic, scientific, and professional workforce.

Cultural Revitalization

By all accounts, our Kanaka 'Ōiwi cultural revival, spurred during the Hawaiian Renaissance of the 1970s, has a strong forward momentum toward further revitalization and integration into Hawai'i's multiethnic society.[29] A vast majority of Kānaka 'Ōiwi (78 to 80 percent) believe it is important to practice and access our culture on a daily basis and for our keiki (children) to learn the Hawaiian language as means of improving cultural pride and developing a positive self-image.[30] Ensuring Ke Ao ʻŌiwi (the Kanaka ʻŌiwi world),[31] the space in society for Kanaka ʻŌiwi culture and people to flourish, is vital to improving the cultural determinants of Mauli Ola.

There are many signs that Kanaka ʻŌiwi culture is thriving: our native language was on the verge of extinction in the early 1980s with only about 1,500 people who spoke the language, predominately kūpuna and Kānaka ʻŌiwi from Niʻihau.[32] Today, it is estimated that about 24,000 people speak our native language, to varying degrees of fluency and across all age groups, because of the proliferation over the past 30 years of Hawaiian language immersion schools, charter schools, and college programs, and kūpuna who are native speakers passing it on to the next generation.[33] Hula, the traditional dance of Hawaiʻi, has also burgeoned in practice since the 1970s so that today there are over 170 hālau hula (hula schools) in Hawaiʻi and 1,100 worldwide.[34] Many Kānaka ʻŌiwi are re-contextualizing ancient social institutions of learning and development for modern applications, such as the Hale Mua (the men's house) and Hale o Papa (the women's house), and revisiting hoʻomana kahiko (ancient forms of empowerment).[35] ʻŌiwi TV, for example, has created the media venue needed to promote the beauty and relevance of our culture to a larger audience. Ke Ao ʻŌiwi is certainly on the rise and helping to improve our social and cultural determinants of Mauli Ola.

This cultural revitalization and integration, coupled with the population increase, can also position Kānaka ʻŌiwi as leaders, not only locally but also among the indigenous world community and other communities concerned with the health of our planet. A good example is the Polynesian Voyaging Society's Mālama Honua Worldwide Voyage, whose mission is to bring awareness to issues, such as global warming and climate change, with the intent of protecting our natural resources and island communities. One of these double-hulled canoes, *Hōkūleʻa,* helped to spur cultural revitalization when, in 1976, it embarked on its maiden voyage to Tahiti. The voyage of *Hōkūleʻa,* along with other voyaging canoes, continues to reinforce the relevance and excellence of Kanaka ʻŌiwi culture with its Mālama Honua Worldwide Voyage. It also demonstrates the role Indigenous Peoples can play in improving the health of the planet because of the values and practices of mālama ʻāina and aloha ʻāina maintained and promoted in our communities.

Participation in the Larger Society

Like the advances and participation we see in promoting the cultural determinants of Mauli Ola, improving social determinants will depend on a similar level of participation by Kānaka ʻŌiwi in the larger society to ensure access to high-quality education, jobs with livable wages, and affordable housing in safe, well-resourced neighborhoods.[36] Education, for example, is an area where the participation of Kānaka 'Ōiwi is vital to Mauli Ola. The Hawai'i public school system does not have a good track record when it comes to educating Kānaka 'Ōiwi, and is likely perpetuating social inequities in Hawai'i.[37] Compared to students of other ethnic groups, Kanaka 'Ōiwi students are more likely to attend low-quality schools with less-experienced teachers, to be overrepresented in special education, to have the highest grade retention rates, and have among the lowest graduation rates[38]—troubling news given that having a good education means a better chance at securing jobs with livable wages and more economic stability.

Because of these education inequities and the lack of cultural relevance, many Kanaka 'Ōiwi leaders and organizations have responded to the need for better educational opportunities for our keiki (children) and 'ōpio (young people) through the creation of culture-based Public Charter Schools and through Kamehameha Schools' Ka Pua Initiative designed to strengthen existing public schools in predominately Native Hawaiian communities. This response by concerned Kanaka 'Ōiwi educators and families to improve the educational situation for Kānaka 'Ōiwi is an example of effective participation in society to improve our collective Mauli Ola. Compared to the performance of Kanaka 'Ōiwi students enrolled in traditional public schools, those enrolled in the culture-based Charter Schools do remarkably better on math and reading tests and have better attendance and engagement with their education.[39] Across both private and public schools, culture-based educational strategies result in Kanaka 'Ōiwi students with greater cultural knowledge and values, stronger Kanaka 'Ōiwi identity, greater emotional and cognitive engagement in their education, and greater sense of place and community and cultural engagement.[40] The culture-based Public Charter Schools and Kamehameha Schools' initiative are excellent examples of how a school system can advance both the social and cultural determinants of Mauli Ola.

Self-Determination and the International Indigenous Movement

During his reign (1874–1891), His Majesty King Kalākaua sought to establish a Polynesian confederation to unite the various nations of the Pacific, in part to ward off European and American imperialism. He was the first head of state to circumnavigate the globe, visiting over twenty nations, to secure the Kingdom of Hawai'i's place among the international community of nations. Despite his efforts, and the efforts of other ali'i (royalty), U.S. imperialism did eventually consume Hawai'i, when in 1893 Her Majesty Queen Lili'uokalani was illegally overthrown by U.S.-supported businessmen, mostly descendants of missionaries. The loss of our nation and the compulsory assimilation strategies and discrimination that followed had a profound deleterious effect on our social and cultural determinants of Mauli Ola.

For many Kānaka 'Ōiwi, achieving self-determination (i.e., the right of a people to freely choose their sovereignty and international political status with no external compulsion or interference)[41] is a strong aspiration because of its potential to expedite the improvement of the social and cultural determinants of Mauli Ola. The degree to which we Kānaka 'Ōiwi can exercise self-determination will influence the impact we can have on these determinants of Mauli Ola, as they are linked social justice issues. Several models of self-determination (e.g., state-within-a-state versus full independence) and the value of U.S. federal recognition as a distinct indigenous U.S. group are debated amongst Kānaka 'Ōiwi[42]—a debate ongoing for over two decades. The eventual settling of this issue of self-determination is vital to our ability to influence our Mauli Ola on our own terms.

The international indigenous movement and the successes achieved in this forum are also important to our self-determination efforts and for facilitating Mauli Ola. Indigenous Peoples throughout the world have sought affirmation of their right to self-determination under international law. In 2007, the United Nations' General Assembly adopted the *Declaration on the Rights of Indigenous Peoples,* which declares entitlement to self-determination.[43] The Declaration refers to the rights of Indigenous Peoples to improve their social and cultural determinants of health, such as education, employment, and housing conditions. It also calls for Indigenous Peoples to decide the manner in which these conditions are addressed. Initially, the United States, along with Australia and New Zealand, were opposed to this declaration citing that "No government can accept the notion of creating different classes of citizens," even though historically these governments intentionally created classes of citizens by forcing indigenous people from their lands and establishing policies that either limited or eliminated their rights as citizens.[44] In 2010, U.S. president Barack Obama, however, placed the United States on the list of 143 countries supporting the Declaration. Although the enforcement of these internationally recognized rights is challenging, to say the least, it does provide a platform for achieving self-determination and protecting our Mauli Ola.

Kanaka 'Ōiwi Aspirations toward Mauli Ola

Kānaka 'Ōiwi, collectively, hold several aspirations important to Mauli Ola as we move into the future, which have also been keys to our resiliency, adaptability, and points for consensus in the past, despite our sociopolitical, socioeconomic, and sociocultural diversity. These aspirations are: 1) the preservation of a strong Kanaka 'Ōiwi identity and the space to assert our perspectives and preferred modes of living, 2) the strengthening of ʻohana values and practices, and 3) the ability to mālama ʻāina and aloha ʻāina.

Kanaka ʻŌiwi Identity and Space

A strong Kanaka ʻŌiwi identity and the physical, emotional, and spiritual space to express this identity (Ke Ao ʻŌiwi) is important to Mauli Ola. Despite over 120 years of U.S. occupation, influx of European and Asian settlers, and compulsory acculturation strategies, 94 to 97 percent of Kānaka ʻŌiwi strongly identify with, and have an affinity toward, their Kānaka ʻŌiwi ancestry and cultural connections.[45] However, researchers have shown how this strong cultural identity might be a source of psychosocial stress for many Kānaka ʻŌiwi because of threats to their identity and preferred modes of living. Kānaka ʻŌiwi with a stronger ethnic identity, for example, perceive more discrimination against them, with about 50 percent reporting frequent instances while the remaining 50 percent report that it occurs "sometimes."[46] Kanaka ʻŌiwi with a stronger cultural identity report more discrimination.[47]

Earlier studies found that Kānaka ʻŌiwi with a stronger identity were more likely to have diabetes, depression, and suicidal behaviors.[48] Subsequent studies found that this may be due to the higher levels of discrimination and cultural discord they experience because of threats to this identity, and that pride (vs. internalization of the discrimination) in one's identity may serve as a buffer against these sources of stress.[49] As indicated earlier, higher levels of perceived discrimination is associated with a higher risk for hypertension and a pattern of cortisol activity associated with heart disease in other populations.

The threats to our identity and their adverse health effects point to changes that need to occur on a larger social and political level. The association between a strong Kanaka ʻŌiwi identity and adverse health outcomes has to do with the experience of greater acculturative stress, discrimination, sense of social injustice, and moral outrage.[50] Kānaka ʻŌiwi with a stronger cultural identity experience more cultural conflict because of living under American influence that does not entirely support our traditional values, practices, and aspirations. The movement to protect Mauna a Wākea on the island of Hawaiʻi from further desecration with the building of the Thirty Meter Telescope (TMT) is a current example of this cultural discord and resulting stress for many Kānaka ʻŌiwi. As our cultural revitalization efforts continue and we assert our Kanaka ʻŌiwi identity and kuleana (prerogatives), these kinds of cultural conflicts and threats are also likely to continue. However, the increase in our population and in Ke Ao ʻŌiwi can provide the critical mass and level of participation necessary to overcome these cultural threats so that we can safely express our indigenous identity and culturally flourish.

Strengthening 'Ohana Relations

An aspiration important to Kanaka 'Ōiwi identity and a means of advancing the positive social and cultural determinants of Mauli Ola is the commitment to 'ohana values and obligations by Kanaka 'Ōiwi families.[51] Compared to other ethnic groups, Kānaka 'Ōiwi are more likely to live in multigenerational households; to have larger 'ohana; to have greater interaction amongst the generations and emotional support; and to have extended 'ohana play a role in child-rearing.[52] 'Ohana values and practices are important sources of resiliency for Kānaka 'Ōiwi, especially for children living in poverty. For example, a Kanaka 'Ōiwi child who believes in the importance of respecting family members and whose parents provide a supportive environment (vs. creating a harsh environment) is less likely to exhibit behavioral problems.[53] These types of 'ohana relations are associated with improved educational outcomes for socially disadvantaged populations.[54]

Aside from ensuring a healthy developmental trajectory for keiki and 'ōpio, strong 'ohana relations can also be important in combating the deleterious effects of discrimination experienced by Kānaka 'Ōiwi. 'Ohana support, coupled with a strong and secure indigenous identity, can lessen the psychological distress caused by discrimination.[55] Most surely, the promotion of these 'ohana values and practices in our young mākua (parents) is necessary to achieving optimal Mauli Ola. They can be promoted and reinforced by culture-based educational strategies applied in our private and public schools and by the many emerging cultural organizations and institutions promoting positive cultural development, such as those previously highlighted.

Ensuring Mālama 'Āina and Aloha 'Āina

Another aspiration important to Kanaka 'Ōiwi identity has to do with mālama 'āina, the ability to care for and cultivate the land to sustain life in perpetuity, and aloha 'āina, the ability to protect and steward the land. The notion of mālama 'āina stems from our mo'okū'auhau (genealogy) and ancestral relations back to Hāloanakalaukapalili (our ancient ancestor) from whom came kalo (our ancient staple food) and its cultivation.[56] The notion of aloha 'āina perhaps came to prominence for Kānaka 'Ōiwi during the time of the overthrow of our kingdom in 1893 as patriotic Kānaka 'Ōiwi fought to restore our Lāhui (Nation), a struggle that continues today. Both mālama 'āina and aloha 'āina continue to be widely practiced and strongly part of the Kanaka 'Ōiwi identity. These are also important issues for the future of our food security (i.e., the availability of enough food to adequately sustain the population) here in Hawai'i, given that 85 to 90 percent of the food we consume is imported.[57]

Kānaka 'Ōiwi are leading the way in addressing our food security while ensuring that we continue to practice mālama 'āina and express aloha 'āina. Some examples include MA'O Organic Farms and Ka'ala Farm in Wai'anae, O'ahu, and Paepae o He'eia in He'eia, O'ahu (a non-profit dedicated to caring for an ancient fishpond). Not only are these Kanaka 'Ōiwi–led farms and fishpond addressing our food and cultural sustainability, they are also providing culture-based education to many keiki and 'ōpio and, in some cases, college opportunities. At the college level recently, a partnership was formed between MA'O Organic Farms, Kamehameha Schools' 'Āina-Based Education Division, and University of Hawai'i (UH) West O'ahu to develop a sustainable community food systems program leading to a Bachelor's of Applied Sciences to prepare students for careers in sustainable food and agriculture sectors in Hawai'i and elsewhere. This partnership is also a good example of how community-based grassroots organizations, Ali'i Legacy organizations, and UH can work collaboratively in improving the social and cultural determinants of Mauli Ola.

Closing Remarks

My intent with this article was to deviate from the usual discourse surrounding the health status of Kānaka 'Ōiwi by moving the focus away from biological factors (e.g., genetic predispositions) and behaviors (e.g., how we eat) to the underlying social and cultural issues that impact our ability to achieve optimal Mauli Ola. Another intent was to highlight the opportunities, strengths, and aspirations of Kānaka 'Ōiwi in advancing our collective Mauli Ola. We have made tremendous advances toward enhancing Mauli Ola over the past forty years. However, whether or not we continue on this path, and the speed by which we travel, will be decided by our actions over the next several decades. Can we rally and find common ground to secure some form of self-governance? Can we apply the same level of participation and resolve given to cultural revitalization toward improving our education and economic situation? Can we leverage our population increase and strong Kanaka 'Ōiwi identity toward regaining social and political capital here in Hawai'i?

Looking thirty years into the future, one of two scenarios is likely to play out. One scenario is the status quo. That is, our mental and physical health status and educational opportunities will continue to be worse than most other ethnic groups in Hawai'i. As our population increases so will the number of Kānaka 'Ōiwi living with chronic diseases and social inequities. Advances in cultural revitalization made over the past forty years will reach a plateau as our attention turns to addressing the overwhelming health needs of the fast-growing Kanaka 'Ōiwi population, made up of predominately young people with limited job opportunities and kūpuna with greater health care needs. Middle-aged Kānaka 'Ōiwi will be challenged with caring for both age groups while struggling to make ends meet. Overall, the status of Ke Ao 'Ōiwi and Mauli Ola will not be too far off from where it is currently, at best.

The other scenario is one in which we as Kānaka 'Ōiwi take advantage of our growing population, cultural revitalization momentum, and civic participation over the next thirty years. In this scenario, Kānaka 'Ōiwi have established Ke Ao 'Ōiwi across all sectors of society and eliminated the harmful effects caused by discrimination here in Hawai'i. Our increased civic participation in the larger society leads to improved systemic changes in education, housing, and wages. We have become leaders in the international indigenous community in indigenous education, cultural revitalization, economic sustainability, and a model of self-governance. As our population increases so does our social and political influence resulting in improvements in our morbidity and mortality rates. Our 'ohana and communities are thriving. Young Kānaka 'Ōiwi are receiving the best education, from both public and private schools, and finding many academic and career opportunities here at home. Kūpuna are not only living longer but healthier so they can enjoy their mo'opuna (grandchildren) and pass on our cultural values, practices, and resiliency. We Kānaka 'Ōiwi have become the population by which all other groups define optimal health and well-being, and we kōkua (help) to bring them along.

Let us work toward the latter scenario. *Kihe, a Mauli Ola!*

NOTES

1. In this chapter, the terms "Kanaka 'Ōiwi" and "Kānaka 'Ōiwi" are used to mean Native Hawaiian (singular) and Native Hawaiians (plural), respectively. Kānaka 'Ōiwi are individuals whose ancestors were the original inhabitants of the Hawaiian archipelago.

2. For a more detailed discussion about the Kapu system in relation to being a public health system, see the article by 'Iwalani R. N. Else, "The Breakdown of the Kapu System and Its Effect on Native Hawaiian Health and Diet," *Hūlili: Multidisciplinary Research on Hawaiian Well-Being* 1, no. 1 (2004): 241–255.

3. These quotes were taken from "The Journals of Captain James Cook on His Voyage of Discovery, vol. III," ed. John Cawte Beaglehole, in *The Voyage of the Resolution and the Discovery, 1776–80* (London: Cambridge University Press, 1968). The first quote is from page 1178 and the second is from page 1181.

4. For a discussion, see Richard Kekuni Blaisdell, "Historical and Cultural Aspects of Native Hawaiian Health," *Social Process in Hawai'i* 32 (1989): 1–21.

5. For more details, see Joseph Keawe'aimoku Kaholokula, "Colonialism, Acculturation and Depression among Kānaka Maoli of Hawai'i," in *Penina Uliuli: Confronting Challenges in Mental Health for Pacific Peoples*, ed. Philip Culbertson, Margaret Nelson Agee, and Cabrini 'Ofa Makasiale (Honolulu: University of Hawai'i Press, 2007); and Marjorie K. Mau, Ka'imi Sinclair, Erin P. Saito, Kau'i N. Baumhofer, and Jo-

seph Keawe'aimoku Kaholokula, "Cardiometabolic Health Disparities in Native Hawaiians and Other Pacific Islanders," *Epidemiologic Reviews* 31 (2009): 113–129.

6. For more information, see Shawn M. Kana'iaupuni, Nolan J. Malone, and Koren Ishibashi, *Income and Poverty among Native Hawaiians: Summary of Ka Huaka'i Findings* (Honolulu: Kamehameha Schools, 2005).

7. These translations of Mauli Ola are from Mary Kawena Pukui and Samuel H. Elbert, *Hawaiian Dictionary: Hawaiian-English*, rev. and enl. ed. (Honolulu: University of Hawai'i Press, 1986).

8. These proverbs and translations are from Mary Kawena Pukui, *'Ōlelo No'eau: Hawaiian Proverbs and Poetical Sayings* (Honolulu: Bishop Museum, 1983), proverbs #1422 and #1788.

9. This definition of health is adapted from the World Health Organization's definition. See http://who.int/about/definition/en/print.html.

10. For more details, see Paula Braveman, Susan Egerter, and David. R. Williams, "The Social Determinants of Health: Coming of Age," *Annual Review of Public Health* 32 (2011): 381–398.

11. For more details, see Francis Mitrou, Martin Cooke, David Lawrence, David Povah, Elena Mobilia, Eric Guimond, and Stephen R. Zubrick, "Gaps in Indigenous Disadvantage Not Closing: A Census Cohort Study of Social Determinants of Health in Australia, Canada, and New Zealand from 1981–2006," *BMC Public Health* 14 (2014): 201.

12. For more details, see Jay S. Kaufman, Lena Dolman, Dinela Rushani, and Richard S. Cooper, "The Contribution of Genomic Research to Explaining Racial Disparities in Cardiovascular Disease: A Systematic Review," *American Journal of Epidemiology* 181, no. 7 (2015): 464–472.

13. For more details, see Catherine Kreatsoulas and Sonia S. Anand, "The Impact of Social Determinants on Cardiovascular Disease," *Canadian Journal of Cardiology* 26, Suppl. C (2010): 8C–13C. Retrieved from http://www.ncbi.nlm.nih.gov/pubmed/20847985.

14. Braveman, Egerter, and Williams, "The Social Determinants of Health: Coming of Age," 381–398.

15. For more discussion, see Mason Durie, "Maori Health: Key Determinants for the Next Twenty-Five Years," *Pacific Health Dialog* 7, no. 1 (March 2000): 6–11; and Shashi Kant, Ilan Vertinsky, Bin Zheng, and Peggy M. Smith, "Social, Cultural, and Land Use Determinants of the Health and Well-Being of Aboriginal Peoples of Canada: A Path Analysis," *Journal of Public Health Policy* 34, no. 3 (2013): 462–476.

16. For more discussion, see Joseph Keawe'aimoku Kaholokula, Andrea H. Nacapoy, and Kā'ohimanu L. Dang, "Social Justice as a Public Health Imperative for Kānaka Maoli," *AlterNative: An International Journal of Indigenous Peoples* 5, no. 2 (2009): 117–137.

17. Historical trauma is also referred to as cultural trauma; it refers to the cumulative emotional and psychological wounding caused by traumatic experiences that extend over an individual's life span that is transmitted from one generation to the next. It is often used to describe the health inequities experienced by indigenous populations in the United States, Canada, New Zealand, and Australia. For more discussion, see Nathaniel Vincent Mohatt, Azure B. Thompson, Nghi D. Thai, and Jacob Kraemer Tebes, "Historical Trauma as Public Narrative: A Conceptual Review of How History Impacts Present-Day Health," *Social Science and Medicine* 106 (2014): 128–136.

18. For more details about this study, see Pallav Pokhrel and Thaddeus A. Herzog,

"Historical Trauma and Substance Use among Native Hawaiian College Students," *American Journal of Health Behavior* 38, no. 3 (2014): 420–429.

19. For more details about these studies, see Joseph Keawe'aimoku Kaholokula, Andrew Grandinetti, Stefan Keller, Andrea H. Nacapoy, Te Kani Kingi, and Marjorie K. Mau, "Association between Perceived Racism and Physiological Stress Indices in Native Hawaiians," *Journal of Behavioral Medicine* 35, no. 1 (2012): 27–37; and Joseph Keawe'aimoku Kaholokula, Marcus K. Iwane, and Andrea H. Nacapoy, "Effects of Perceived Racism and Acculturation on Hypertension in Native Hawaiians," *Hawai'i Medical Journal* 69, no. 5, Suppl. 2 (2010): 11–15.

20. For more detail about this study, see Van M. Ta, Puihan J. Chao, and Joseph Keawe'aimoku Kaholokula, "Cultural Identity and Conceptualization of Depression among Native Hawaiian Women," *AAPI Nexus Journal: Policy, Practice, and Community* 8, no. 2 (2010): 63–85.

21. These are population estimates from Kamehameha Schools, *Ka Huaka'i 2014: Native Hawaiian Educational Assessment* (Honolulu: Kamehameha Schools, 2014), 17.

22. This assertion is based on past and current patterns in longevity between ethnic groups in Hawai'i. For more details about longevity across ethnic groups in Hawai'i, see Chai Bin Park, Kathryn L. Braun, Brian Y. Horiuchi, Caryn Tottori, and Alvin. T. Onaka, "Longevity Disparities in Multiethnic Hawaii: An Analysis of 2000 Life Tables," *Public Health Reports* 124, no. 4 (2009): 579–584.

23. Kamehameha Schools, *Ka Huaka'i 2014*, 251.

24. Numerous studies have linked lower educational attainment to higher morbidity and mortality. For one example of these studies, see Cameron A. Mustard, Shelley Derksen, Jean-Marie Berthelot, Michael Wolfson, and Leslie L. Roos, "Age-Specific Education and Income Gradients in Morbidity and Mortality in a Canadian Province," *Social Science & Medicine* 45, no. 3 (1997): 383–397.

25. For more details about this demographic study, see the article by Sara Kehaulani Goo, "After 200 Years, Native Hawaiians Make a Comeback," Pew Research Center (2015), published electronically April 6, 2015, at http://www.pewresearch.org/fact-tank/2015/04/06/native-hawaiian-population/. Her article is based on David Swanson's study, "A New Estimate of the Native Hawaiian Population for 1778, the Year of First European Contact."

26. For an excellent discussion on how infectious diseases decimated the Kanaka 'Ōiwi population from the late 1700s to early 1900s, see Ozzie A. Bushnell, *The Gifts of Civilization: Germs and Genocide in Hawai'i* (Honolulu: University of Hawai'i Press, 1993).

27. For a review of diabetes, heart disease, and their risk factors in Kānaka 'Ōiwi, also see Mau, Sinclair, Saito, Baumhofer, and Kaholokula, "Cardiometabolic Health Disparities in Native Hawaiians and Other Pacific Islanders," 113–129.

28. This estimate is based on data from the Department of Business, Economic Development and Tourism reported in *Population and Economic Projections for the State of Hawai'i to 2040* (Honolulu: State of Hawai'i Department of Business, Economic Development and Tourism, 2012), which can be obtained at http://files.hawaii.gov/dbedt/economic/data_reports/2040-long-range-forecast/2040-long-range-forecast.pdf.

29. This is actually considered the second Hawaiian Renaissance. The first was during Kalākaua's reign (1883–1891), in which he reinstituted traditional Hawaiian practices previously banned, such as hula, chants, and other rituals. The second is believed to have its roots in the 1970s with the resurgence of Hawaiian music and lan-

guage, hula, and the return of ancient navigation, and in the many land struggles of the time.

30. Kamehameha Schools, *Ka Huaka'i 2014*.

31. The term Ke Ao 'Ōiwi is used here to refer to the space and place needed for Kānaka 'Ōiwi to flourish. It refers to the idea that optimum health of Kānaka 'Ōiwi can only be achieved in a society that values their social group and provides the sociocultural space for their preferred modes of living and aspirations. For more discussion, see Joseph Keawe'aimoku Kaholokula, "Achieving Social and Health Equity in Hawai'i," in *The Value of Hawai'i 2: Ancestral Roots, Oceanic Visions*, ed. Aiko Yamashiro and Noelani N. Goodyear-Ka'opua (Honolulu: University of Hawai'i Press, 2014).

32. Hawaiian language revitalization was spurred by concerns over the small number of native and fluent speakers who, by the 1980s, were mostly Kūpuna and persons from Ni'ihau. 'Aha Pūnana Leo website provides a Hawaiian language revitalization time line. See http://www.ahapunanaleo.org/index.php?/about/a_timeline_of_revitalization/.

33. This estimate is based on data from the US Census, "Table 1. Detailed Languages Spoken at Home and Ability to Speak English for the Population 5 Years and over for the United States: 2006–2008," in *American Community Survey Data on Language Use* (Washington, DC: US Census Bureau, 2010).

34. This estimate is based on information provided on mele.com in its "Hālau Hula Listing."

35. For an example of ancient institutions being revitalized, see the article by Samson Reiny, "A Kane in Full," *Hana Hou!* (October/November 2013).

36. Sir Mason Durie is a respected Māori leader known for his contributions to Māori health. He has written extensively on the key determinants of Māori health, one of which is participation by Māori in the larger society. For more discussion, see Mason Durie, *Nga Kahui Pou: Launching Maori Futures* (Wellington, NZ: Huia, 2003), 292.

37. Jonathon Y. Okamura, in chapter 4 of his book *Ethnicity and Inequality in Hawai'i* (Philadelphia: Temple University Press, 2008), provides an analysis of the educational inequities perpetuated by the public school system in Hawai'i.

38. For more details, see Shawn M. Kana'iaupuni and Koren Ishibashi, *Left Behind? The Status of Hawaiian Students in Hawai'i Public Schools* (Honolulu: Kamehameha Schools, 2003).

39. For more details, see Shawn M. Kana'iaupuni and Koren Ishibashi, *Hawai'i Charter Schools: Initial Trends and Select Outcomes for Native Hawaiian Students*, PASE Report (Honolulu: Kamehameha Schools, 2005).

40. More details can be found in a series of 2009 reports (Hawaiian Cultural Influences in Education) prepared by Brandon Ledward and Brennan Takayama at http://www.ksbe.edu/spi/cbe_findings/. See bibliography for their full citations.

41. For a broader discussion of self-determination, see Jeff J. Corntassel and Tomas Hopkins Primeau, "Indigenous 'Sovereignty' and International Law: Revised Strategies for Pursuing 'Self-determination,'" *Hawaiian Journal of Law & Politics* 2 (2006): 52–72.

42. For diverse Kanaka 'Ōiwi perspectives on self-determination and discussions on Hawaiian movements, see Noelani Goodyear-Ka'opua, Ikaika Hussey, and Erin Kahunawaika'ala Wright, eds., *A Nation Rising: Hawaiian Movements for Life, Land, and Sovereignty* (Durham, NC: Duke University Press, 2014). For another perspective on Hawaiian sovereignty, see David Keanu Sai, *Ua Mau Ke Ea—Sovereignty Endures: An*

Overview of the Political and Legal History of the Hawaiian Islands (Honolulu: Pūʻā Foundation, 2011).

43. For more discussion, see "United Nations Declaration on the Rights of Indigenous Peoples," adopted by the United Nations General Assembly on September 13, 2007, which can be obtained at http://www.un.org/esa/socdev/unpfii/documents/DRIPS_en.pdf.

44. For more discussion, see Anup Shah, "The Rights of Indigenous People" (2010). Retrieved from Global Issues: Social, Political, Economic and Environmental Issues That Affect Us All, http://www.globalissues.org/article/693/rights-of-indigenous-people#MajorCountriesOpposedtoVariousRightsforIndigenousPeoples.

45. This assertion is based on several studies examining the relationship between Kanaka ʻŌiwi identity and certain health statuses. For a discussion of these studies, see Joseph Keaweʻaimoku Kaholokula, Andrea H. Nacapoy, and Kāʻohimanu L. Dang, "Social Justice as a Public Health Imperative for Kānaka Maoli," *AlterNative: An International Journal of Indigenous Peoples* 5, no. 2 (2009): 117–137. For a discussion on the effects of cultural identity on the mental health of Kanaka ʻŌiwi women, see Van M. Ta, Puihan Chao, and Joseph Keaweʻaimoku Kaholokula, "Cultural Identity and Conceptualization of Depression among Native Hawaiian Women," *AAPI Nexus Journal: Policy, Practice, and Community* 8, no. 2 (2010): 63–85.

46. For more details, see previously noted Kaholokula et al. (2009, 2012) articles.

47. For more details, see previously noted Kaholokula et al. (2012) article.

48. For more details about these studies, see previously noted articles by Kaholokula et al. (2008) and Kaholokula (2007), and article by Noelle Y. C. Yuen, Linda B. Nahulu, Earl S. Hishinuma, and Robin. H. Miyamoto, "Cultural Identification and Attempted Suicide in Native Hawaiian Adolescents," *Journal of the American Academy of Child Adolescent Psychiatry* 39, no. 3 (2000): 360–367.

49. These assertions are based on research findings detailed by Kaholokula et al. (2009) and Pokhrel and Herzog (2014). Their citations were previously noted.

50. For more discussion on the psychological factors affecting health outcomes in Kānaka ʻŌiwi, see previously noted articles by Kaholokula (2007) and Ta et al. (2010). Also see William C. Rezentes, *Ka Lama Kukui—Hawaiian Psychology: An Introduction* (Honolulu: ʻAʻaliʻi Books, 1996).

51. For a broader discussion on identity and ʻohana, see Shawn M. Kanaʻiaupuni, "Identity and Diversity in Contemporary Hawaiian Families: Hoʻi Hou I Ka Iwi Kuamoʻo," *Hūlili: Multidisciplinary Research on Hawaiian Well-Being* 1 (2004): 53–71.

52. These assertions are made based on works by Deborah Goebert et al. (2000), Shawn Kanaʻiaupuni et al. (2005), and Ivette Rodriguez Stern, Sylvia Yuen, and Marcia Hartsock (2004). See bibliography for full citations.

53. For more details, see previously noted article by Kaholokula et al. (2009) and article by Barbara D. DeBaryshe, Sylvia Yuen, Lana N. Nakamura, and Ivette R. Stern, "The Role of Family Obligations and Parenting Practices in Explaining the Well-Being of Native Hawaiian Adolescents Living in Poverty," *Hūlili: Multidisciplinary Research on Hawaiian Well-Being* 3, no. 1 (2006): 103–125.

54. For more details see Andrew J. Fuligni, "Family Obligation and the Academic Motivation of Adolescents from Asian, Latin American, and European Backgrounds," *New Directions for Child Adolescent Development*, no. 94 (Winter 2001): 61–75.

55. For more details, see Meifen Wei, Christine Jean Yeh, Ruth Chu-Lien Chao, Stephanie Carrera, and Jenny C. Su, "Family Support, Self-Esteem, and Perceived Ra-

cial Discrimination among Asian American Male College Students," *Journal of Counseling Psychology* 60, no. 3 (July 2013): 453–461.

56. Hāloanakalaukapalili (Long stem-shaky-leaf-trembling) was the child of Wākea (sky father) and Ho'ohokuikalani (daughter of Wākea) who was born abnormal. He was buried outside the house of Wākea and from this site the first kalo grew. Wākea and Ho'ohokuikalani went on to have another child who was named Hāloa in honor of his elder brother—the ancestor of the Kanaka 'Ōiwi race.

57. For more discussion, see Office of Planning report, "Increased Food Security and Food Self-Sufficiency Strategy," edited by Economic Development and Tourism Department of Business (Honolulu: State of Hawai'i, 2012). The report can be obtained from http://files.hawaii.gov/dbedt/op/spb/INCREASED_FOOD_SECURITY_AND_FOOD_SELF_SUFFICIENCY_STRATEGY.pdf.

BIBLIOGRAPHY

Beaglehole, John Cawte, ed. "The Journals of Captain James Cook on His Voyage of Discovery." *The Voyage of the Resolution and the Discovery, 1776–80,* vol. III. London: Cambridge University Press, 1967.

Blaisdell, Richard K. "Historical and Cultural Aspects of Native Hawaiian Health." *Social Process in Hawai'i* 32 (1989): 1–21.

Braveman, Paula, Susan Egerter, and David R. Williams. "The Social Determinants of Health: Coming of Age." *Annual Rev Public Health* 32 (2011): 381–398.

Bushnell, Ozzie. A. *The Gifts of Civilization: Germs and Genocide in Hawai'i.* Honolulu: University of Hawai'i Press, 1993.

Corntassel, Jeff J., and Tomas H. Primeau. "Indigenous 'Sovereignty' and International Law: Revised Strategies for Pursuing 'Self-Determination.'" *Hawaiian Journal of Law & Politics* 2 (2006): 52–72.

DeBaryshe, Barbara D., Sylvia Yuen, Lana N. Nakamura, and Ivette R. Stern. "The Role of Family Obligations and Parenting Practices in Explaining the Well-Being of Native Hawaiian Adolescents Living in Poverty." *Hūlili: Multidisciplinary Research on Hawaiian Well-Being* 3, no. 1 (2006): 103–125.

Department of Business, Economic Development and Tourism. *Population and Economic Projections for the State of Hawaii to 2040.* Honolulu: Department of Business, Economic Development and Tourism, 2012.

Durie, Mason. "Maori Health: Key Determinants for the Next Twenty-five Years." *Pac Health Dialog* 7, no. 1 (March 2000): 6–11.

———. *Nga Kahui Pou: Launching Maori Futures.* Wellington, NZ: Huia, 2003.

Else, 'Iwalani R. N. "The Breakdown of the Kapu System and Its Effect on Native Hawaiian Health and Diet." *Hūlili: Multidisciplinary Research on Hawaiian Well-Being* 1, no. 1 (2004): 241–255.

Fuligni, Andrew J. "Family Obligation and the Academic Motivation of Adolescents from Asian, Latin American, and European Backgrounds." *New Directions for Child and Adolescent Development,* no. 94 (Winter 2001): 61–75.

Goebert, Deborah, Linda Nahulu, Earl Hishinuma, Cathy Bell, Noelle Yuen, Barry Carlton, Naleen N. Andrade, Robin Miyamoto, and Ronald Johnson. "Cumulative

Effect of Family Environment on Psychiatric Symptomatology among Multiethnic Adolescents." *Journal of Adolescent Health* 27, no. 1 (July 2000): 34–42.

Goo, S. "After 200 Years, Native Hawaiians Make a Comeback." Pew Research Center (2015). Published electronically April 6, 2015. http://www.pewresearch.org/fact-tank/2015/04/06/native-hawaiian-population/.

Goodyear-Ka'opua, Noelani, Ikaika Hussey, and Erin Kahunawaika'ala Wright, eds. *A Nation Rising: Hawaiian Movements for Life, Land, and Sovereignty*. Narrating Native Histories. Durham, NC: Duke University Press, 2014.

Kaholokula, Joseph Keawe'aimoku. "Colonialism, Acculturation and Depression among Kānaka Maoli of Hawai'i." In *Penina Uliuli: Confronting Challenges in Mental Health for Pacific Peoples*, ed. P. Culbertson, M. N. Agee, and C. Makasiale. Honolulu: University of Hawai'i Press, 2007.

Kaholokula, Joseph Keawe'aimoku, Andrew Grandinetti, Stephan Keller, Andrea H. Nacapoy, Te Kani Kingi, and Marjorie K. Mau. "Association between Perceived Racism and Physiological Stress Indices in Native Hawaiians." *Journal of Behavioral Medicine* 35, no. 1 (February 2012): 27–37.

Kaholokula, Joseph Keawe'aimoku, Marcus K. Iwane, and Andrea H. Nacapoy. "Effects of Perceived Racism and Acculturation on Hypertension in Native Hawaiians." *Hawai'i Medical Journal* 69, no. 5, Suppl. 2 (May 2010): 11–15.

Kaholokula, Joseph Keawe'aimoku, Andrea H. Nacapoy, and Kā'ohimanu L. Dang. "Social Justice as a Public Health Imperative for Kānaka Maoli." *AlterNative: An International Journal of Indigenous Peoples* 5, no. 2 (2009): 117–137.

Kaholokula, Joseph Keawe'aimoku, Andrea H. Nacapoy, Andrew Grandinetti, and Healani K. Chang. "Association between Acculturation Modes and Type 2 Diabetes among Native Hawaiians." *Diabetes Care* 31, no. 4 (April 2008): 698–700.

Kamehameha Schools. *Ka Huaka'i 2014 Native Hawaiian Educational Assessment*. Honolulu: Kamehameha Schools, 2014.

Kana'iaupuni, Shawn M. "Identity and Diversity in Contemporary Hawaiian Families: Ho'i hou i ka iwi kuamo'o." *Hūlili: Multidisciplinary Research on Hawaiian Well-Being* 1 (2004): 53–71.

Kana'iaupuni, Shawn M., and Koren Ishibashi. *Hawai'i Charter Schools: Initial Trends and Select Outcomes for Native Hawaiian Students*. PASE Report. Honolulu: PASE (Policy Analysis & System Evaluation), Kamehameha Schools, 2005.

———. *Left Behind? The Status of Hawaiian Students in Hawai'i Public Schools*. Honolulu: Kamehameha Schools, 2003.

Kana'iaupuni, Shawn M., Nolan J. Malone, and Koren Ishibashi. *Income and Poverty among Native Hawaiians: Summary of Ka Huaka'i Findings*. Honolulu: Kamehameha Schools, 2005.

———. *Ka Huaka'i: 2005 Native Hawaiian Educational Assessment*. Honolulu: Kamehameha Schools, 2005.

Kant, Shashi, Ilan Vertinsky, Bin Zheng, and Peggy M. Smith. "Social, Cultural, and Land Use Determinants of the Health and Well-Being of Aboriginal Peoples of Canada: A Path Analysis." *Journal of Public Health Policy* 34, no. 3 (August 2013): 462–476.

Kaufman, Jay S., Lena Dolman, Dinela Rushani, and Richard S. Cooper. "The Contribution of Genomic Research to Explaining Racial Disparities in Cardiovascular Disease: A Systematic Review." *American Journal of Epidemiology* 181, no. 7 (April 1, 2015): 464–472.

Kreatsoulas, Catherine, and Sonia S. Anand. "The Impact of Social Determinants on Cardiovascular Disease." *Canadian Journal of Cardiology* 26 Suppl. C (August–September 2010): 8C–13C.

Ledward, Brandon, and Brennan Takayama. *Hawaiian Cultural Influences in Education (HCIE): Community Attachment and Giveback among Hawaiian Students.* Honolulu: Kamehameha Schools, 2009.

———. *Hawaiian Cultural Influences in Education (HCIE): Cultural Knowledge and Practice among Hawaiian Students.* Honolulu: Kamehameha Schools, 2009.

Mau, Marjorie K., Ka'imi Sinclair, Erin P. Saito, Kau'i N. Baumhofer, and Joseph Keawe'aimoku Kaholokula. "Cardiometabolic Health Disparities in Native Hawaiians and Other Pacific Islanders." *Epidemiologic Reviews* 31 (2009): 113–129.

Mele.com. "Halau Hula (Hula Schools)." 2010.

Mitrou, Francis, Martin Cooke, David Lawrence, David Povah, Elena Mobilia, Eric Guimond, and Stephan R. Zubrick. "Gaps in Indigenous Disadvantage Not Closing: A Census Cohort Study of Social Determinants of Health in Australia, Canada, and New Zealand from 1981–2006." *BMC Public Health* 14 (2014): 201.

Mohatt, Nathaniel Vincent, Azure B. Thompson, Nghi D. Thai, and Jacob K. Tebes. "Historical Trauma as Public Narrative: A Conceptual Review of How History Impacts Present-Day Health." *Social Science & Medicine* 106 (April 2014): 128–136.

Mustard, Cameron A., Shelley Derksen, Jean-Marie M. Berthelot, Michael Wolfson, and Leslie L. Roos. "Age-Specific Education and Income Gradients in Morbidity and Mortality in a Canadian Province." *Social Science & Medicine* 45, no. 3 (August 1997): 383–397.

Okamura, Jonathan Y. *Ethnicity and Inequality in Hawai'i.* Philadelphia: Temple University Press, 2008.

Park, Chai Bin, Kathryn L. Braun, Brian Y. Horiuchi, Caryn Tottori, and Alvin T. Onaka. "Longevity Disparities in Multiethnic Hawaii: An Analysis of 2000 Life Tables." *Public Health Reports* 124, no. 4 (July–August 2009): 579–584.

Pokhrel, Pallav, and Thaddeus A. Herzog. "Historical Trauma and Substance Use among Native Hawaiian College Students." *American Journal of Health Behavior* 38, no. 3 (May 2014): 420–429.

Pukui, Mary Kawena, and Samuel H. Elbert. *Hawaiian Dictionary: Hawaiian-English, English-Hawaiian.* Rev. and enl. ed. Honolulu: University of Hawai'i Press, 1991.

Reiny, Samson. "A Kane in Full." *Hana Hou Magazine,* October–November 2013.

Rezentes, William C. *Ka Lama Kukui—Hawaiian Psychology: An Introduction.* Honolulu: 'A'ali'i Books, 1996.

Sai, David Keanu. *Ua Mau Ke Ea—Sovereignty Endures: An Overview of the Political and Legal History of the Hawaiian Islands.* Honolulu: Pū'ā Foundation, 2011.

Shah, Anup. "The Rights of Indigenous People." Published electronically October

16, 2010. http://www.globalissues.org/article/693/rights-of-indigenous-people#MajorCountriesOpposedtoVariousRightsforIndigenousPeoples.

State of Hawai'i, Office of Planning. "Increased Food Security and Food Self-sufficiency Strategy." Edited by Economic Development and Tourism Department of Business. Honolulu: State of Hawai'i, 2012.

Stern, Ivette R., Sylvia Yuen, and Marcia Hartsock. "A Macro Portrait of Hawaiian Families." *Hūlili: Multidiscplinary Research on Hawaiian Well-Being* 1, no. 1 (2004): 73-92.

Ta, Van M., Puihan Chao, and Joseph Keawe'aimoku Kaholokula. "Cultural Identity and Conceptualization of Depression among Native Hawaiian Women." *AAPI Nexus Journal: Policy, Practice, and Community* 8, no. 2 (2010): 63–85.

Takayama, Brennon, and Brandon Ledward. *Hawaiian Cultural Influences in Education (HCIE): Positive Self-Concept*. Honolulu: Kamehameha Schools, 2009.

———. *Hawaiian Cultural Influences in Education (HCIE): School Engagement among Hawaiian Students*. Honolulu: Kamehameha Schools, 2009.

United Nations, General Assembly, Office of the High Commissioner for Human Rights. United Nations Declaration on the Rights of Indigenous Peoples: Adopted by the General Assembly on September 13, 2007. Pocket-sized format ed. New York: OHCHR, 2008.

US Census. "Table 1. Detailed Languages Spoken at Home and Ability to Speak English for the Population 5 Years and Over for the United States: 2006–2008." In *American Community Survey Data on Language Use*. Washington, DC: US Census Bureau, 2010.

Wei, Meifen, Christine Jean Yeh, Ruth Chu-Lien Chao, Stephanie Carrera, and Jenny C. Su. "Family Support, Self-Esteem, and Perceived Racial Discrimination among Asian American Male College Students." *Journal of Counseling Psychology* 60, no. 3 (July 2013): 453–461.

Yuen, Noelle Y., Linda B. Nahulu, Earl S. Hishinuma, and Robin H. Miyamoto. "Cultural Identification and Attempted Suicide in Native Hawaiian Adolescents." *Journal of the American Academy of Child and Adolescent Psychiatry* 39, no. 3 (March 2000): 360–367.

E Ola Mau: Insights on Pathways to Health

Richard Kekuni Blaisdell, Mele A. Look, Kamuela Werner, and Benjamin Young

Esteemed kupuna and founding faculty of the University of Hawai'i's John A. Burns School of Medicine, Dr. Richard Kekuni Blaisdell was the first oral history interview for the school's Native Hawaiian Center of Excellence's Oral Video History Project developed by then Center of Excellence director Dr. Benjamin Young. The purpose of this watershed project was to record the career pathways of notable Native Hawaiians into science and medicine. This video collection of sixteen oral history interviews is available through the University of Hawai'i at Mānoa libraries. Kekuni Blaisdell has been an essential presence in two pivotal areas of Native Hawaiian well-being, which he believes are intrinsically connected: Hawaiian political sovereignty and improvement of Native Hawaiian health status. He was an early and outspoken leader in both areas during times when these issues were unpopular and frequently dismissed. His courage, aloha, and perseverance in bringing attention to these concerns through public, personal, and professional means endeared him to legions of activists, physicians, patients, and students.

Kekuni Blaisdell's interview was conducted in 2000 at his family home in Nu'uanu, O'ahu, under the guidance of the film's producer, Nanette Napoleon, and director, Heidi Chang. In 2015, a transcription of the interview was completed and proofed by two independent readers from the medical school's Department of Native Hawaiian Health for accuracy and completeness. To facilitate a narrative style, a thematic methodology was then used to identify subject areas. Three department members independently read the transcript and assigned topic areas to the text. Then notes were compared to reach unanimous agreement on the frequency of each thematic area. The text was then reorganized under respective themes. The questions were eliminated and text was inserted using brackets to aid readability. The manuscript's text was minimally edited and notes added to enhance clarity of conversational style. Kekuni Blaisdell, with assistance from his daughter Dr. Nalani Blaisdell, made additional edits upon final review; these changes from the original transcript have been noted.

Being Kanaka Maoli

Aloha kipa mai i ku'u home o Kaohinani. Maika'i ikaika nā hau'oli i loko nei e 'ike i kou maka. Welcome to our home.

I am *Kanaka Maoli*[1] and it was very clear as a youngster that I was. I was treated like one but lived in a *haole*[2] dominated world and the message from my parents and grandparents was to act like a haole in order to survive.[3] When I graduated from Kamehameha Schools, I identified myself in the yearbook not as "Kekuni," but as "Dick Blaisdell" because that was what I felt was an acceptable and suitable haole name.

Kanaka means a human being, a person. Maoli means true, real, genuine, and coming from the 'āina, the land, which is being part of our sacred environment. That is the way our ancestors identified themselves when the first foreigners came so that is the way we identify ourselves. When I was a youngster, the term Kanaka was usually a term of derision and an unpleasant, pejorative adjective associated with it such as "dirty Kanaka," "lazy Kanaka," "drunken Kanaka," or "dumb Kanaka." That was why we use the term now, Kanaka Maoli, meaning we are as our ancestors were.[4]

One of my students, Dr. Emmett Aluli,[5] was in the Kānaka Maoli rights movement right from the beginning while he was a medical student, and I remember wondering, *"What is this young man up to? He should decide if he is going to be a doctor or an activist."* It was not until 1980 that I became aware of the plight of our people. In 1983, I was asked to participate in preparing the Native Hawaiian Study Commission Report[6] created by the United States Congress. I discovered what I had not known before; we Kānaka Maoli had the worst health indicators of all ethnic peoples in our homeland as well as the worst social, economic, and educational indicators. Therefore, there must be underlying root causes in need of proper attention if we were going to do something about it. About that time, I was approached by three longtime activists, Soli Kihei Niheu, Puhipau, and Imaikalani Kalahele, to join the movement for independence. After reflecting on this, I made the commitment. That is how I came into the movement, committed to *kūoko'a*, independence of our homeland. We consider our sovereignty to mean independence—there is no other model because anything less means dependence. We consider kūoko'a, independence, to be the natural state of man and dependence to be unnatural.

Living a Healthy and Fulfilling Life

[Living a healthy and fulfilling life is part of] the Kānaka Maoli philosophy, which stems from clear and strong self-identity as Kānaka Maoli. It is being in constant communication and relationship with our ancestors who continue to be with us in this current temporal world in many forms such as *Wākea,* our sky father, and *Papa,* our earth mother. By our own basic anatomy, we are constantly reminded of three important connections. So, we have three *piko.*[7] Most people know about the *piko waena,* the central piko or point, which is the navel, the remnant of each person's individual attachment during intrauterine life with his or her mama by which the fetus and the embryo receives nutrients from the placenta and the uterus in the womb of each person's mother. The gut is the *nā'au,* the seat of learning, wisdom, and feeling. "Gut feeling" refers to that kind of knowledge. According to our own traditional concepts, we have not learned anything unless we can feel it and act on it. Learning is much more than just memorizing words and passing a written examination. The second piko is the *manawa,* or the *piko po'o* in the skull. In the infant, it is the anterior fontanel connecting the personal *'uhane*[8] or *wailua* with our ancestors all the way back to the beginning of time. As long as we think, listen, and talk about them, and are guided by them, we are connected. The third piko is the *piko ma'i,* between the legs. That connects us with our *mamo,* our descendants after us forever! Therefore, we do not have a linear relationship but a timeless circular one. Those are the basic beliefs; because of those, how can we despair? How can we lack confidence or self-esteem, and begin to neglect and abuse ourselves, or others in our family? It is because we have forgotten who we are. By returning to those basic, simple, and yet strong traditional beliefs, values, and concepts as Kānaka Maoli we care not only for ourselves but with all—*I kekahi i kekahi.*[9]

Hawaiian Concepts of Health and Medicine

The concepts of Hawaiian medicine are basic concepts to our culture and way of life. They really stem from "*'O ke ao i ka huli wela ka honua, o ke ao i ka lole ka lani.*" Those are the opening lines of *He Kumulipo,*[10] and it really provides the basic concepts of Kanaka Maoli thought and cosmic view and therefore the basis of life and healing. The opening lines refer to the hot earth turning against the changing skies and that is the metaphor for Papa, earth mother, mating with Wākea, sky father. Out of that mating comes everything in our cosmos, and since we all have the same parents that means that we are all *'ohana,* and since our parents are living that means that everything in our cosmos is living, conscious, and also communicating. This is very different from the dominant Western view, which distinguishes between that which is living—animate—and that which is not living—inanimate. In the Kanaka Maoli world, everything is living: the wind, the sounds, the lights, the shadows, the rocks, and the waters. Everything is living and we as Kānaka Maoli are 'ohana to all of this from the beginning of time. We are just temporarily here and after us comes our mamo which continues this life and connects with our ancestors. We consider life to be timeless and not linear, but circular. Spirituality is the basis for our cosmic view of life and therefore as to how illness comes about and how it needs to be prevented and treated.

[Kānaka Maoli] did not practice medicine in the sense that we think, because in daily living they practiced prevention of mishaps, misfortunes—including illness. Part of growing up as a youngster was learning how to do this for oneself and becoming caring for one self. The basic foods, for example, were preventives. *Lapa'au*[11] is not merely taking care of oneself or others when one is ill. Lapa'au means also *hō'ola,* and that is making health and promoting health by preventing illness. We do that every time we say the proper prayers, have the proper thoughts and images while incorporating these important staples.

Lā'au lapa'au refers to the use of plants as medicine. We use these plants to remain well and free of illness. There are also lā'au but not medicine in the Western sense, that is, taking medicine in order to get over an illness. We are taking lā'au to remain healthy and prevent being ill. Illness in pre-Western times, according to writings and chants, came about because of some imbalance—a disharmony between the person individually—because of something the person did or did not do, or perhaps because of some harmful influence outside of the person. This diminished the individual's *mana* and that is why the person became ill. Therefore, the approach was to determine what was this factor within oneself. Was it because of something one had done? Some offense against oneself or someone else that was responsible for this? Or did it come from outside? You had to find out. Upon finding out, one corrected this. Self-diagnosis began by the person asking those questions and beginning to make amends. It is only if one remains sick and couldn't deal with it adequately that one went, usually to the elder within the family, who was trained and gifted. One would have to explain and the elder would help to take care of the problem. Only when the illness persisted, and if one could afford to, one went to the *heiau hō'ola*—the temple of healing. If there was one nearby; one came under the care of the *kahuna lā'au lapa'au*—one of the specialized medical practitioners. These were the kahuna[12] who maintained these special healing temples where they treated people who had serious illnesses that could not be taken care of by other means. Usually they took care of chiefs for example. There they also engaged in research and learning about medicinal properties of plants. They also trained younger *haumana,* students, to become eventually kahuna lapa'au. That was the system of old as described by several subsequent writers such as Samuel Kamakau.[13]

I am not really qualified to practice [Hawaiian traditional medicine]. I still consider myself a student. There are aspects to Hawaiian medicine, most people are aware of lā'au—the use of Hawaiian medicinal plants, that's difficult and very complicated. I am still learning. Another technique is, of course, *lomilomi*,[14] and I love to lomilomi so I never hesitate to do that even informally. But I'm still trying to learn the skill of *kāhea*,[15] which is "calling." I consider myself a neophyte and officially certified and licensed only to practice Western medicine.

In 1999 [I was part of a group] to actually conduct the [first] course at the University of Hawai'i at Mānoa on lapa'au. Lapa'au is a broad term that covers the Hawaiian medicine with all of the specialties. Fortunately, the school of public health—which existed at that time, through Professor John Caskin—proposed such a course. Professor Caskin asked me to coordinate the course, bringing together suitable specialists to conduct it during the summer in July of 1999 at the University of Hawai'i at Mānoa at the Center for Hawaiian Studies. We were very grateful to the School of Public Health and University Center for Hawaiian Studies for providing the opportunity for us to do that as well as the practitioners in the community who contributed to teaching.

Native Hawaiians in Medicine

It was my job [when I came to the University and they were initially developing the medical school] to establish a Department of Medicine. We started as a two-year medical school, our Department of Medicine was the only clinical department. All others were non-clinical: anatomy, biochemistry, physiology, microbiology, pharmacology, and pathology. Our task was to prepare our two-year medical students for acceptance in four-year medical schools on the continental United States without any serious handicap or difficulty during their start. It was a serious challenge because third-year students take not only medicine but surgery, psychiatry, pediatrics, obstetrics, and gynecology. Therefore, our Department of Medicine had to engage those major clinical specialties to provide at least beginning, basic fundamental experiences so that when they moved into those clinical rotations on the continent they would be able to perform. Our first class graduated in 1975. In that class we had four notable Kānaka Maoli graduates who already made very prominent imprints in relieving the plight of our people. One is Noa Emmett Aluli of Protect Kaho'olawe prominence, also a physician on Moloka'i. Another is Dr. William Ahuna, who pioneered cultural competency among physicians in the Kaiser system. The third is Nathan Wong, also with the Kaiser system and also, like Dr. Benjamin Young,[16] a crewmember on the *Hōkūle'a*.[17] The fourth is Dr. Solomon Naluai, who practiced public health medicine.[18]

Initially, I was the only full-time Kanaka Maoli member of the faculty. Part-time faculty, physicians in practice who served as faculty, included Dr. George Mills. Dr. George Mills was very prominent in the Hawai'i Medical Associa-

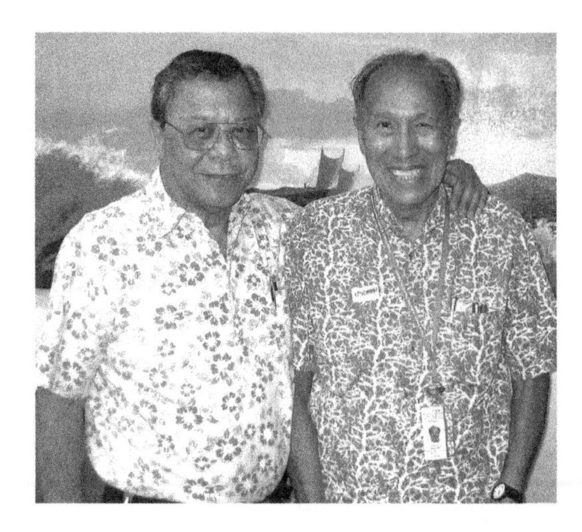

Figure 3.1. Drs. Kekuni Blaisdell and Benjamin Young at the Bishop Museum, 2010. Photo by Chace Moleta, used with permission.

tion and was the longtime president of the Hawaiian Civic Clubs. Dr. Allen Richardson was an orthopedic surgeon and also president of the Hawai'i Medical Association. His son, Allen Richardson, was the chief of orthopedic surgery in the Department of Surgery in our medical school. Dr. Charman Akina, Kanaka Maoli physician with the Medical Group, also served as physician at Waimānalo Community Health Center. We are very proud of those pioneering Kānaka Maoli physicians.

[When I was growing up, the Native Hawaiian physician] I most remember was Alexander Kaonohi, a naturopathic physician who had a large practice in Kapahulu. He used not only modern Western medicine but also some traditional Hawaiian medical methods. Papa Ola Lokahi, the Native Hawaiian coordinating health organization created by the United States Congress, honors Dr. Alexander Kaonohi by its Alexander Kaonohi awards that are given to people who have contributed to Native Hawaiian health. I was honored to be one of those recipients.

Medical Career Pathways

There is desperate need [for Kānaka Maoli to pursue medicine]. We Kānaka Maoli have the worst health, economic, social, educational indicators of all ethnicities in our homeland. The United States Congress projects that in the year 2040 there will be no more Kānaka Maoli.[19] We are all 'ohana, therefore we have an obligation, *kuleana,* responsibility to care for each other and to share with each other. That is what we have to do. It is not a matter of option—there are no options. We have to do it if we are Kānaka Maoli.

The Native Hawaiian Center of Excellence, whose [former] director is Benjamin Young, recruits and encourages more Kānaka Maoli to enter health pro-

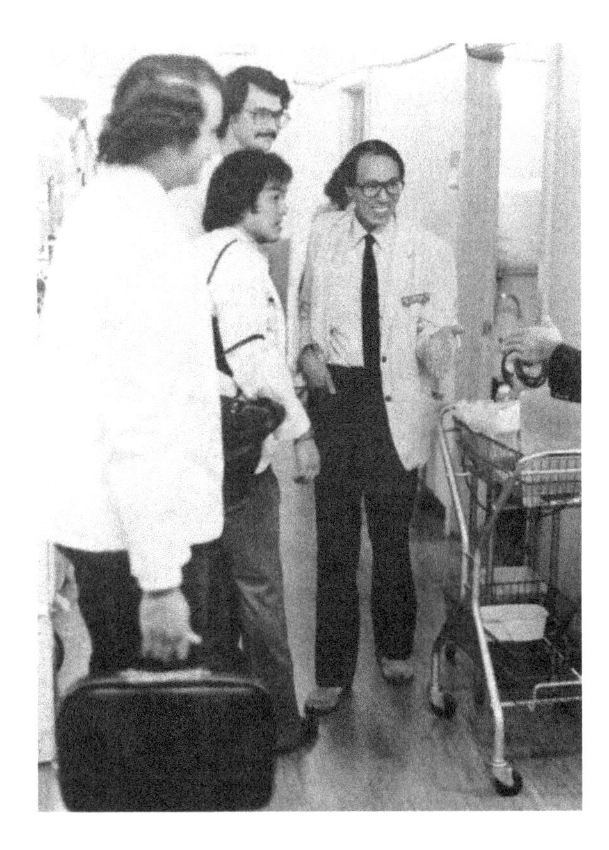

Figure 3.2. Dr. Kekuni Blaisdell and medical students, 1975. Photo courtesy of JABSOM, used with permission.

fessions in order to lead the grave health needs of our people. We have the worst health statistics, highest mortality rates for major causes of death such as heart disease, cancer, stroke, and diabetes. The highest morbidity rates such as hypertension, diabetes, heart failure, and coronary heart disease, also the highest rates for complications of pregnancy. Also, the highest suicide rates, but it's not confined to just health, we also have the highest rates for dropout from the public schools.

Medical education currently is case-based, that is, problem case-based. Beginning in the first year, they learn biochemistry, anatomy, physiology, and pharmacology in relationship to particular cases in what they call PBL cases.[20] Then every week, these are first-year students now, they meet with a clinical preceptor such as myself in the hospital or in a clinical setting and see patients that illustrate the kind of PBL cases they are having in their tutorials in problem-based-learning. That is very different from the conventional or traditional medical education that I had in my day even though at that time when I went to medical school it was considered a reformed curriculum. At that time, there were two years in the pre-clinical basic sciences such as anatomy and chemistry and at the end of the second year we began to see patients. We would be prepared to take care of sick patients in the third and fourth year. But in our medical school when we started in 1966 with the first class, our students began to see patients the first week, once a week. They were in the hospital with white coats and with their instruments talking with and examining patients.

I talk to my students about "*'elima mea nui,*" which is five important things. The first one is the patient comes first—not the doctor, not the nurse, not the hospital, not the medical school, not the student, but the patient. It is a privilege that society gives us to serve as physicians to patients. That has to be paramount in whatever we do and though it sort of seems obvious it is sometimes very difficult but one has to always keep it in mind realizing that sometimes we violate that cardinal principle. The second is that doctor, the term doctor, means teacher, and therefore it's also essential that we continue to learn to teach ourselves to learn from patients, learn from our colleagues, and learn from our medical students so that we are constantly right at the cutting edge of knowledge and skills in caring for our patients. The third refers to bringing science to the bedside. Science ordinarily refers to Western science based on the scientific method which is based on evidence. There is nothing that we should do in caring for patients that isn't based on evidence. Fourth, is to have fun, to enjoy what we're doing because if we aren't enjoying what we are doing no matter how difficult and how tired we are then maybe we should consider something else to do. And the fifth mea nui, important thing, is that we are at a special place. Our homeland of *Ka Pae 'Āina*[21] is a special place, no other like it and this is a special time that we are here together learning how to take care of sick people, and therefore we must be special. There must be a reason, there must be a purpose, and it is for us to work out what that is.

My Pathway into Medicine

The curriculum[22] at the Kamehameha Schools for boys, at that time the lower campus where the Bishop Museum is now, was a military school and the curriculum focused on what was called industrial arts. I was training to be an electrician, and the curriculum had an extra year. We had seventh, eighth, ninth, tenth, and then low eleventh and high eleventh, and then the senior grades. Twelfth grade and the high eleventh, senior boys every two weeks worked somewhere in town. I worked as an electrician at what was then Hawaiian Pine—what is now Dole Company, as an electrician.

One of the teachers was Donald Kilolani Mitchell. We called him Kilolani, which means observer of the heavens, because he liked to teach us about the stars and he became our science teacher at the old campus. He suggested that I consider going into medicine, and I talked it over with my parents and decided that we would take a try at it. That is how it happened. When I left Kamehameha, I was accepted at the University of Redlands in California. The war was on at that time. I graduated in 1942 and went to the University of Redlands in California till 1944.

[The University of Chicago School of Medicine was where I selected to go because] the president of the university at that time was Robert Maynard Hutchins.[23] He became president of the university at the age of 30. He came to the university from a position of dean of the Yale Law School and had created a whole new reform educational movement, reforming the educational system so that it was based on critical thinking and on studying the classics. He created with Professor Mortimer Adler "the great books curriculum." It was through his influence that I first learned about the University of Chicago and then discovered that they had a top ranking medical school. In fact, just before I went, they had two medical schools, University of Chicago–School of Medicine on the south side and Rush Medical College on the west side. That is why I went there. The University of Chicago was the first medical school to have an entirely full-time faculty and university hospital right on the campus as part of the university with all of the patients. It was a school devoted to research, education, and training. Not only physicians to practice but also to teach and to pursue research. I felt very honored.

Within the university, I didn't have any difficulty [adjusting], on the other hand when I went to find a new place to live in a private home, I was turned away when the landlady discovered that I was not white, and although I had a name Blaisdell, she told me that she did not accept anyone who was not white. I know what racism is. My mother got me started [in the payment for medical school]. My mother always worked and my father, of course, later became fire chief. Before he had married my mother, he had a previous family of three children, but it was mainly my mother who continued to work until she died while I was in medical school who got me started. I always worked while at the University of Redlands and also at the University of Chicago. At Chicago for example, I worked as a dishwasher in the girls' dormitory. I got my meals free and that relieved me of considerable expense.

[I was] thrilled, exhilarated, when I was accepted for the Osler internship at the Johns Hopkins Hospital![24] Johns Hopkins Hospital was a pioneer in medical education and also research. I was very honored. William Osler[25] was a Canadian. Prior to his time, medical students learned medicine not in the hospitals but in the lecture halls. He pioneered at Johns Hopkins by putting medical students right in the hospital—taking care and learning from sick patients. We had no pay at all but we were provided living quarters, meals, and uniforms. We were on every night, seven days a week, and had only one week vacation.

After my year at Johns Hopkins, I went south to Tulane in New Orleans and was a medical resident there at Charity Hospital. Johns Hopkins is in the south too, and racism was very blatant in both of those institutions. For example, at Johns Hopkins there were separate restrooms for "colored" people and white people. The blood bank had separate blood for white people and "colored" people, and it was the same at Charity Hospital in New Orleans. Charity Hospital was divided right down the middle. Separate entrances on the east for "colored" people and on the west for white people and separate blood in blood banks. I was on the Tulane medical service at Charity Hospital for one year.

The Korean War was on [at that time] and I knew that I was going to be drafted. In order to anticipate that, I volunteered and was in the regular army for four years—initially assigned to the Quarter Master Climatic Research Laboratory in Lawrence, Massachusetts. I lived in Andover, which is nearby, this was north and not too far from Boston. I was in the research laboratory there but had an opportunity to become familiar with the medical institutions in Boston such as Harvard Medical School and Brigham Hospital. I had a classmate from the University of Chicago at Massachusetts General Hospital who later became chief of surgery—John Holman's Professor of Surgery. That is Paul Russell, who was my classmate at the University of Chicago.

After four years in the army, I went to Duke [University Hospital] for a year in pathology and that was arranged for me by Professor Wiley Forbes. He was a consultant to the MAG Formosa; the Military Assistance and Advisory Group on the Island of Taiwan, which was called Formosa at that time. I completed medical residency with two more years at the University of Chicago and had a fellowship in hematology. That's how I became a hematologist. Not only an internist but a hematologist—that is a blood specialist.

There are two main reasons [that I became interested in hematology]. One, I was inspired by the professor and chief of hematology there, Dr. Leon Jacobson, who had pioneered in the use of isotopes in medicine and hematology as the chief consultant to the Manhattan Project, which was the atomic bomb research project at the University of Chicago. I was also very attracted by these beautiful, colorful blood cells. These cells took on special color developed by stains developed by Dr. Paul Ehrlich in Europe in the previous century. That's how I became a hematologist.

One of my early heroes was [my Kamehameha School science teacher] Kilolani Mitchell, when I was in medical school I liked to teach and decided at that time I would try to become a full-time academician. Although I knew it was a very difficult track and knew I might not be able to make it. At that time, I began to think about it and through my internship and residency experiences I was able to become a member of the faculty at the University of Chicago. Through that position I was invited to become a professor of medicine and to start the Department of Medicine at what is now the John A. Burns School of Medicine of the University of Hawai'i.[26]

Medical Research and Humanity

[From 1959 to 1961 I was chief of hematology for the Atomic Bomb Casualty Commission in Hiroshima and Nagasaki, which] came about through Franklin McLean,[27] who was the first professor of medicine and chairman of the Department of Medicine at the University of Chicago. In the late 1950s, when I had returned to the University of Chicago, Franklin McLean had retired officially as a professor of medicine. He was a first-rate researcher in bone metabolism and had a research laboratory in the Department of Physiology. He was prominent as a researcher and well known in Washington as a consultant to the National Academy of Sciences, which is part of the government. It had responsibility for establishing the atomic bomb casualty commission in Hiroshima and Nagasaki after the Second World War. He told me that the atomic bomb casualty commission was looking for a hematologist and suggested I look into it. That is how that came to be. I was there for two years and lived in a small fishing village of Mogimachi outside of Nagasaki. I took a bus everyday into the Nagasaki Atomic Bomb Casualty Commission and, when needed, would take the overnight train to Hiroshima.

My role was to conduct research on the survivors, the *hibakusha,* atomic bomb survivors who had been exposed to nuclear radiation. As most people know, even before I went there, an alarming rate of leukemia began to appear in these survivors. It was one of my jobs to follow up on the occurrence not only of leukemia, but of other blood disorders, such as so called aplastic anemia or marrow failure, a blood disorder that is similar to leukemia but not overt leukemia. We also discovered at that time a peculiar prevalence of leukopenia "low white count" which we were never really able to explain in the atomic bomb survivors. That is the kind of research we did or I did when I was in both Nagasaki and Hiroshima. We saw atomic bomb survivors every day. It was a part of the program to examine and follow them and see what else developed. Besides those disorders, other types of cancers such as thyroid cancer began to be detected in those survivors. I learned that it is very different when one lives among and with the people who have been exposed to such devastation and to be identified with a country that was responsible for that. That is one of the reasons why I am anti-nuclear and anti-military and pro-peace through justice.

Family History

My full name is Richard Kekuni Akana Blaisdell. Kekuni comes from my father's family. My father was James Akana, and his mother was a Wongham and his grandmother a Keli'ikipi from the Island of Maui. The name Kekuni comes from that family, "Keli'ikipi from Maui." Kekuni refers to a fire ceremony that was used by a special division of kahuna. *"Kuni"* was a ceremony using fire to define the nature of an illness so that the illness could be properly treated. Presumably, somewhere in my family there was a *kahuna kuni* and that is how the name came to be. I was born in 1925 on March 11 in the old Kapi'olani maternity hall. I grew up in Kaimukī on Pāhoa Avenue.

My father was James Kealiikauahi Akana, but his father was Paul Yim, who was born in Canton. He was an immigrant and my father was one of I believe 10 children born on Ohua Lane. My father and his siblings were born there because the Queen [Lili'uokalani] provided a home for my father's mother, my grandmother whose name was Martha Akiau Wongham Yim Akana. She was a servant in the household of the Queen.

My mother was Margarite Nameleonalani Piltz and her father,[28] Captain George Piltz, was captain of the *Dickinson,* the cable ship successive to the *Florence Ward.* The sailing ship helped to lay the cable between the west coast of the United States to here and then Japan. Captain George Piltz married my grandmother, Mariah Pu'uohau.[29] She was an orphan. She and her siblings became orphaned at a very young age. Their parents were in the household of Princess Miriam Likelike. Her parents were Thomas and Priscilla Pu'uohau in the household of Princess Miriam Likelike. When she [the princess] died, her older sister, Lili'uokalani, took the children into her home and sent them to school.[30] One of them was my grandmother, Mariah, and she married Captain George Piltz. They had six children and my mother was the oldest living of those children. We were very, very close as a family and so I had Kanaka Maoli 'ohana who lived in Waikīkī near where the queen lived. We were very close to that Pu'uohau and Kaeo family. The Kaeo family also married the Ka'awakauwo family. We were brought up together as Kānaka Maoli. I learned the importance of sharing, giving, loving, and the importance of being close to nature. On the other hand, my parents and my grandparent were Christians so we were brought up to be Christians and this "kahuna-ism" was considered the work of the devil. So it was not until later that I began to appreciate the importance of our own Kanaka Maoli religion, what the haoles called "kahuna-ism."

I was in the second grade at Punahou School when my father died at the age of 39 of peritonitis complicating ruptured appendix. I was without a father at that very critical tender age. My mother remarried in 1940, William Blaisdell, who later became fire chief. I was fortunate to have a second father [and he was also] the brother of Neal Blaisdell. Mayor Neal Blaisdell who was number one son and the second son was William Blaisdell. So that's how I acquired the name Blaisdell. I was hanai by William Blaisdell.

[When I was living in Japan I adopted my son], at that time I was still a bachelor, unmarried and one of my colleagues in the Department of Pathology and his wife had just adopted a youngster although they had two children of their own. There were orphans in Japan, and there was a professor, a retired professor at the local university there who had taken upon himself to arrange adoptions by foreigners, such as Americans, for Japanese youngsters who didn't have a home. So, I learned through that experience how to do it and I was able to find Mitsunori, who became Mitsunori Kamakani[31,32] Blaisdell. When I adopted him officially, even though I was a single parent at that time, I was able to find *obasan*[33] Eguchisan to take care of him at our little house in Mogimachi, outside of Nagasaki. So he was a little over a year of age, and then when I returned to the University of Chicago I had a son. After two years in Chicago, I found a wife who became the mother to my son. My wife was Irene Saito, who was a Waimānalo plantation girl and was a nurse at the University of Chicago.[34] And so our son, Mitsunori, was one of the best men at our wedding in the Catholic Church, Saint Thomas Church in Chicago, on the south side of Chicago. Then we had a daughter, Nalani Blaisdell,[35] who was born at the University of Chicago, Chicago Lying-In Hospital. [In 1966] the four of us came to Hawai'i. [I am very proud of the fact that] my wife was a nurse and of course my daughter, Nalani Blaisdell, graduated from the John A. Burns School of Medicine in 1999.

He mea iki 'ia. Mahalo iā 'oe no kēia manawa, kēia ha'i 'ōlelo no au e pili ana nā mea o nā mea a mau, a mau.

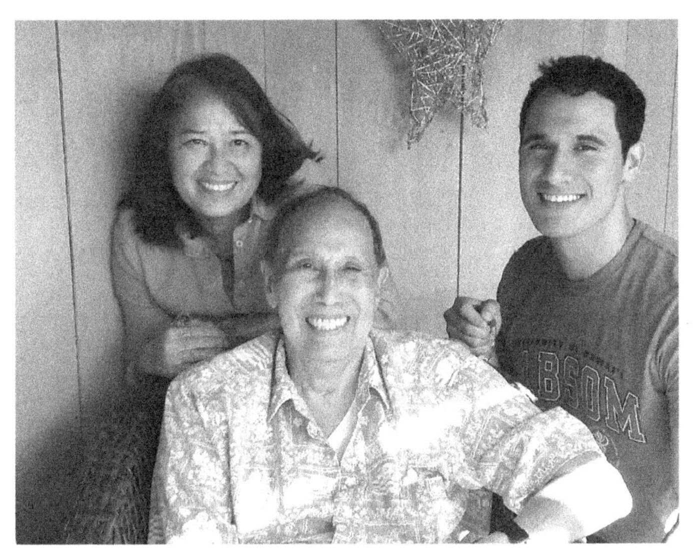

Figure 3.3. Dr. Kekuni Blaisdell, Mele Look, and Kamuela Werner at his Nu'uanu residence, 2014. Photo courtesy of Mele Look, used with permission.

Mahalo piha and aloha are extended to Nalani Blaisdell, Nanette Napoleon, and Heidi Chang. Appreciation for funding support is extended to The Queen's Health Systems, National Institute of Minority Health and Health Disparities (P20MD000173), and the Health Resources and Services Administration of the U.S. Department of Health and Human Services under the University of Hawai'i Native Hawaiian Center of Excellence (D34HP16044). The content is solely the responsibility of the authors and does not necessarily represent the official views of its funders.

NOTES

1. In Kekuni Blaisdell's lecture notes from August 11, 2009, he noted that British seaman Archibald Campbell's book *A Voyage Round the World, From 1806–1812,* published by Duke & Browne in London, 1822, reported that people of Sandwich Islands (Hawai'i) call themselves "Cannakamowree" (Kanaka Maoli).

2. Pukui and Elbert, *Hawaiian Dictionary,* 58: white person, American, Englishman, or Caucasian; any foreigner.

3. Original text, "so I was ashamed to be Kanaka" was removed upon request by N. Blaisdell and R. K. Blaisdell, July 11, 2015.

4. Original text, "I am a late comer [to the Kānaka Maoli sovereignty movement]" was removed upon request by N. Blaisdell and R. K. Blaisdell, July 11, 2015.

5. Noa Emmett Aluli, MD, was one of six Native Hawaiians in the first graduating class of the John A. Burns School of Medicine in 1975. While still in medical school he became a renowned leader of the Protect Kaho'olawe 'Ohana grassroots organization that led the political activism of the 1970s to stop the U.S. Navy from using the island for target practice, an activity that began in World War II. After decades of protests, court battles, and clean-up efforts, Kaho'olawe was returned to state in 1993 and its management is overseen by the Kahoolawe Island Reserve Commission, of which Protect Kaho'olawe 'Ohana is a member.

6. The Native Hawaiian Study Commission's purpose was to conduct a study of the culture, needs, and concerns of Native Hawaiians. A majority and minority report was submitted to Congress. The Minority Report, issued on June 23, 1983, stated the United States was morally responsible for the overthrow of the monarchy.

7. Pukui and Elbert, *Hawaiian Dictionary,* 328: navel, navel string, or umbilical cord; figuratively used to describe blood relative, and genitals.

8. Ibid., 363: soul, spirit, or ghost.

9. Ibid., 142: "I kekahi i kekahi," meaning to one or the other, alternatingly.

10. Kumulipo is the name of a Hawaiian creation chant, and Kekuni Blaisdell has noted that he frequently conferred with scholar Rubellite Kawena Johnson on interpretation of the Kumulipo.

11. Pukui and Elbert, *Hawaiian Dictionary,* 194: medical practice; to treat with medicine, heal, or cure.

12. Ibid., 114: priest, sorcerer, magician, wizard, minister, and an expert in any profession including medicine. In the 1845 Kingdom of Hawai'i's laws doctors, surgeons, and dentists were called kahuna.

13. Samuel Kamakau was a prominent Native Hawaiian scholar of the nineteenth

century. Kamakau collected and published his research on the history and traditions of his people.

14. Pukui and Elbert, *Hawaiian Dictionary*, 212: to squeeze and chafe the limbs of one who is weary or in pain. This massage modality is one of the traditional Native Hawaiian healing practices still utilized in contemporary times.

15. *Kāhea* is defined as a Native Hawaiian traditional healing modality based on use of prayer, literally, "to call."

16. Benjamin Young, MD, is the first Native Hawaiian psychiatrist. At the University of Hawai'i Medical School, he served as associate dean of students as well as director of the Native Hawaiian Center of Excellence. He established the 'Imi Ho'ōla Post-Baccalaureate Program and was a founding member and early leader of the Polynesian Voyaging Society.

17. *Hōkūle'a*, meaning clear star or star of gladness, is the name of a double-hulled voyaging canoe built and launched in the 1970s by the Polynesian Voyaging Society. This sea vessel and its crew were instrumental in changing scientific understanding of Polynesian migratory history and symbolized renewed pride in Pacific Islanders' heritage as oceanic voyagers.

18. The four Hawaiian physicians identified were part of the Dean's Guest Program, a predecessor to the current 'Imi Ho'ōla Program. Two additional Hawaiian physicians were in that inaugural class: Bruce Nelson, MD, and Richard Ching, MD. Both had prominent careers and made notable contributions.

19. In a technical report issued as part of the Native Hawaiian Health Care Act of 1993, the full-blooded Native Hawaiian population numbers were reported to be declining and that by 2040 the population count for this group would be too small to be considered a separate population.

20. Problem-based learning (PBL) is defined as an educational methodology utilizing small-group discussions of clinical cases as the stimulus for learning.

21. Pukui and Elbert, *Hawaiian Dictionary*, 394: group of islands or archipelago.

22. Original text, "[My pursuit of a medical career] was an aberration because the official curriculum [at Kamehameha Schools] was for us, Kanaka Maoli, to be trained to be blue collar workers to serve the industry, at that time which was mainly sugar and pineapple. That was the ceiling, and there really was not an official college preparation course. All of the faculty was haole, white people fresh off the boat from the continental United States. Their task was to bleach us, to make white men out of us, at least in mind set," was removed upon request by N. Blaisdell and R. K. Blaisdell, July 11, 2015.

23. Also known as Maynard Hutchins (January 17, 1899–May 17, 1977), he was an American educational philosopher, dean of Yale Law School (1927–1929), and president (1929–1945) and chancellor (1945–1951) of the University of Chicago. While he was president of the University of Chicago, Hutchins implemented wide-ranging and controversial reforms at the university, including the elimination of varsity football. The most far-reaching reforms involved the undergraduate college of the University of Chicago, which was retooled into a novel pedagogical system built on great books, Socratic dialogue, comprehensive examinations, and early entrance to college.

24. Kekuni Blaisdell was the first Native Hawaiian to receive this prestigious medical internship.

25. Sir William Osler, 1st Baronet (July 12, 1849–December 29, 1919), was a Canadian physician and one of the four founding professors of Johns Hopkins Hospital.

Osler created the first residency program for specialty training of physicians, and he was the first to bring medical students out of the lecture hall for bedside clinical training. He has frequently been described as "the father of modern medicine."

26. Kekuni Blaisdell was the first Native Hawaiian to chair a department of medicine in a U.S. medical school.

27. Dr. Franklin Chambers McLean (1888–September 10, 1968) was a professor and chairman of the Department of Medicine and the first appointed director of the University of Chicago Medical Clinics, as well as the founder of the National Medical Fellowships. He aided the Manhattan Project by studying the effects of radiation on organisms. He was also a trustee of the Julius Rosenwald Fund as well as Fisk University.

28. Original text, "was a haole," was removed upon request by N. Blaisdell and R. K. Blaisdell, July 11, 2015.

29. Both Mariah Pu'uohau and Martha Akiau Wongham Yim Akana were *piha* or full Hawaiian in blood quantum.

30. Queen Lili'uokalani hānai[-ed] these children. Hānai is a Hawaiian practice defined as adoption, foster, raise, rear, feed, nourish, sustain.

31. Original text, "Kamakanika'ilialoha," was replaced by "Kamakani" upon request by N. Blaisdell and R. K. Blaisdell, July 11, 2015.

32. Mitsunori Kamakani Blaisdell is his legal name, and his full Hawaiian name given by his father, Kekuni Blaisdell, is Kamakanika'ilialoha, translated as the love-snatching-wind and also the title to a well-known Hawaiian song, "Ka Makani Kā'ili Aloha," with its poignant refrain, *"Ku'u pua, ku'u lei, ku'u milimili ē/Ku'u lei kau i ka wēkiu/A he milimili 'oe a he hiwahiwa na'u/A he lei mau no ku'u kino,"* translated as "My flower, my lei, mine to cherish/My lei that I adore above all others/You are my favorite and precious to me/A lei forever for my body." Source: Charles E. King, *King's Book of Hawaiian Melodies* (Miami Beach: Hansen House, 1948), 28. Personal communication to M. Look, March 27, 2001.

33. Seigo, *Japanese-English English-Japanese Dictionary*, 172: aunt.

34. Irene Saito Blaisdell graduated from St. Francis School in Mānoa and the University of Washington School of Nursing in Seattle.

35. Helen Kaleleonalani Blaisdell is her full given name. Kaleleonālani is translated as the-flight-of-the-heavenly-ones.

BIBLIOGRAPHY

Nakao, Seigo. *Japanese-English English-Japanese Dictionary.* New York: Random House, Inc., 1997.

Pukui, Mary Kawena, and Samuel H. Elbert. *Hawaiian Dictionary: Hawaiian-English, English-Hawaiian.* Rev. and enl. ed. Honolulu: University of Hawai'i Press, 1986.

He Lama ʻĀ Hoʻokahi
Mele Inoa for Dr. Richard Kekuni Blaisdell

Joseph Keaweʻaimoku Kaholokula

He Lama...
He Lama ʻā hoʻokahi
I Kapālama, mai Kilolani
He kilohana ka ʻike ʻia ʻana
O ka Lama kū o ka loea

He Lāʻau...
He Lāʻau kū hoʻokahi
He muʻo, he kupu, e ulu aʻe
Paʻa ka mole i ke one hānau
He lau, he lālā, he kumu paʻa

He Lehua...
He Lehua uʻi hoʻokahi
Paʻapū ʻia aku i ke kahua
He kumu muimuia i ka manu
I ka waonahele, i uka, i Nuʻuanu

He Alakaʻi...
He Alakaʻi kaʻi hoʻokahi
Mai moku Keawe a Kahelelani
He pouhana nui o ka hale,
Mai nā kūpuna ke koʻo paʻa

He Leo...
He Leo hea hoʻokahi
Wawā ʻia ka Lāhui i Hawaiʻi
He lono i ke kāhea
Heahea akula, e ʻonipaʻa

He Kanaka...
He Kanaka hano hoʻokahi
Nui ke alo, Haʻahaʻa ke ʻano

He aloha nui aku ʻia nā pōkiʻi
I Waokanaka ka noho ʻana

E Ola...
E ola! E ola! E ola mau e!
No ka hanohano o Kekuni!

An enlightenment...
A torch burning like no other
In Kapālama, from Kilolani
A desire for learning was sparked
A path to excellence was undertaken

A tree [also reference to medicine]...
A tree [Dr.] that stands like no other
A bud, a shoot, growing forth
Until his roots were firmly planted in his birth sands
A leaf, a branch, a mature tree now stands strong

An expert [especially warrior]...
An expert with beauty like no other
The foundation has been covered with many Lehua
A fine Lehua tree that attracts many birds
In the forest, in the uplands, in Nuʻuanu

A leader...
A leader that leads like no other
From Hawaii to Kauai
He is like a center post that keeps the house standing
From our ancestors comes his strength to do so

A voice...
A voice that beckons like no other
His voice echoes throughout our Nation
A call goes out
He calls to all to stand firm

A man...
A man who distinguishes himself like no other
Enormous is his presence, but humble is his demeanor

A great admiration is bestowed upon him by all
In Waokanaka he resides

Live . . .
Live, live, live long!
It is said in honor of Kekuni!

Mele inoa composed for the inaugural Kekuni Blaisdell Lectureship at the John A. Burns School of Medicine at the University of Hawai'i, 2007.

ʻImi Hoʻōla: Reflections of Dreams Come True

Kelli-Ann Frank Voloch, Karen K. Sakamoto, Patrice Ming-Lei Tim Sing, Nanette Kapulani Mossman Judd, Akolea K. Ioane, and Leimomi Noel Kanagusuku

This is about dreams that come true for those who remain steadfast and believe in serving others. The ʻImi Hoʻōla Post-Baccalaureate Program seeks to improve health care in Hawaiʻi and the Pacific by increasing the number of physicians committed to practicing in underserved communities and producing a more diverse health-care workforce. ʻImi Hoʻōla has forty years of experience guiding underrepresented students to prepare for and complete the medical degree program at the John A. Burns School of Medicine (JABSOM) at the University of Hawaiʻi. The twelve-month educational program addresses students' academic and professional needs and focuses on their strengths and weaknesses in order to develop self-directed, lifelong learners. The program encourages students to develop their critical thinking skills through the use of a problem-based learning approach with the objective of producing service-oriented medical leaders.

Established in 1972 by Dean Windsor Cutting, the ʻImi Hoʻōla program recruited fifteen students. Classes began in 1973 under Dean Terence A. Rogers at a time when there were only ten physicians of Hawaiian ancestry in Hawaiʻi. Initially a pre-medical enrichment program, ʻImi Hoʻōla became a post-baccalaureate program in 1996, offering provisional acceptance to medical school at JABSOM to socially, economically, and/or educationally disadvantaged students. Founding director Benjamin B. C. Young, MD, sought counsel from Mary Kawena Pukui, the late Hawaiian writer and scholar, to help name the program. The words *ʻimi* (seek) and *hoʻōla* (heal) were chosen and the program was named ʻImi Hoʻōla (Those who seek to heal). Up to twelve students are now enrolled in the program each year and, upon successful completion of the program, enter JABSOM as first-year medical students.

The success of ʻImi Hoʻōla is best illuminated through a close examination of its outcomes. In this case, those outcomes shine through the brief profile presented here on Nanette Judd, PhD, RN. Dr. Judd is professor emeritus and retired program coordinator and director of ʻImi Hoʻōla, having served for more than thirty years. Following Dr. Judd's incredible story are the dreams of success and reflections of graduates of the 'Imi Ho'ōla program currently enrolled at JABSOM as well as those practicing in various communities of Hawai'i.

Nanette Judd, Professor Emeritus and Former Director, 'Imi Ho'ōla Post-Baccalaureate Program

After more than thirty years, Nanette Judd is still shaping the lives of those she has mentored. Since childhood, Nanette Kapulani Mossman Judd knew she was destined to pursue a career in health care through the encouragement of her grandparents, parents, and extended family. Her mother and aunt were both registered nurses and now her own son has chosen the same noble cause! Nanette fondly remembers the *mo'olelo* (stories) told by her late mother, Violet Kiope Beazley Mossman, about her father, who was a soldier in the Spanish-American War. He was well cared for by nurses after being injured while serving in the U.S. Navy. The stories told conveyed gratitude for the Navy nurses who tended to him, helping him to recover and later raise a family. He urged his young daughters to become nurses, and two of them did exactly that.

Nanette's place in the family tree is as the eldest daughter and second child of a Christian Hawaiian family, born and raised on the island of O'ahu. She continues to live on O'ahu, happily married to Donald Wayne Judd, and is a mother of two sons, Michael and Boyd, and a grandmother of a thriving 'ohana with *mo'opuna* (grandchildren) to whom she passes on *mana'o* (wisdom) and love. "Growing up, I had the role model of my own mother," she says, "so when 'ohana or others would ask me what I would grow up to be, I would tell

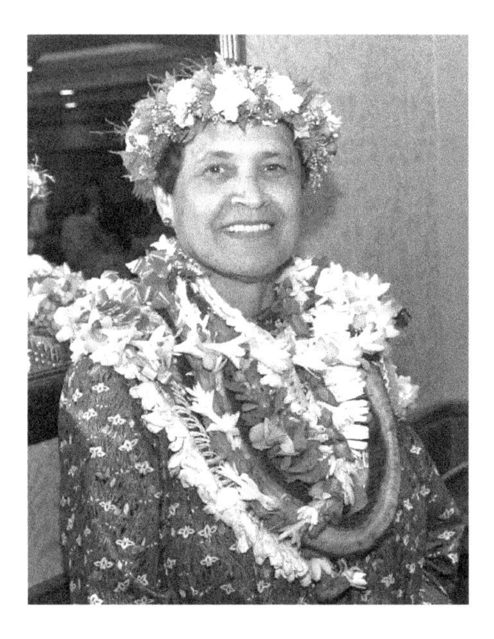

Figure 5.1 Dr. Nanette Judd, retired program coordinator and director of 'Imi Ho'ōla. Photo courtesy of Kelli-Ann Voloch.

them, 'go ask my mother!' " Her mother would often say, "You can take *it* anywhere and no one can take *it* away from you!" The operative term of "it" being education, and in particular, health care education. Nanette's mother greatly influenced her chosen career as a public health nurse. After graduating from the Kamehameha Schools Kapālama campus in 1962, she pursued a bachelor of nursing degree and a public health nurse certificate from the University of California at Chico and graduated in 1966. Soon after, Nanette married, and both she and her husband chose to serve as Peace Corps volunteers. She proudly recalls answering the charge of President John F. Kennedy: "...ask not what your country can do for you but what you can do for your country."

Their Peace Corp group trained for three months on the island of Moloka'i before duty, living an immersion-style existence. They were required to learn to speak the Pohnpeian dialect via their local guides and lived in tents to practice a minimalist lifestyle in isolation. They learned how to build a latrine and shower as well as other subsistence shelters. When they arrived in Pohnpei in the remote archipelago of Micronesia, Nanette functioned as the public health nurse for the community. Nurse Judd gave immunizations, collected Hansen's disease data, and provided routine family health care and education. The group worked together to figure out how to navigate through the newly experienced and wonderful Micronesian culture. To this day, Nanette continues to be amazed at how similar the local people were to her own family and culture. Pohnpeians wanted to be healthy, parents wished for a better life for their children, and all were proud of their own culture and values.

As a young nurse, Nanette began seeing firsthand how different levels of lifestyle affected people. The socioeconomic divides, educational differences and deficiencies, as well as poorer health standards—such as lack of clean water—changed the potentials and possibilities for families and communities. These scenarios served as the impetus for the growth of her lifelong work with those who, through no fault of their own, found themselves in a disadvantaged position but sought to improve their lives. Nanette began to emerge as a leader and advocate in the fight for health-care equality. Many have been privileged to receive just that, leadership and advocacy, simply by meeting her.

Several pivotal learning opportunities occurred during Nanette's volunteer work in Micronesia and the lessons learned were instrumental in her lifelong work for social justice. Her philosophy of optimism—not the rose-colored glasses kind, but the one that sparks solution-based change around a communal force for good—has been central to every step and decision in her career path. She calls it the "do the right thing attitude." Nanette chose a profession in nursing with the hope of moving masses of people toward a healthier life via direct care, but also with policy change and referral processes as a public health–trained provider. Nurse Nanette began her career seeing the need to make a positive difference on a tiny island archipelago in the Pacific. She went on to do more from a broader platform with 'Imi Ho'ōla by guiding hundreds of disadvantaged students on their journey to become doctors.

Another important realization for Nanette that began in Micronesia was the power of being a change agent if it was predicated by a shared worldview. As a public health nurse there was health education to share with her Pohnpeian families, sometimes involving the need to change the way they collected their water, or cooked, or cleaned, or other things that potentially increased their illness risk. Nanette was often the bridge between the Western way of doing things and the local people's way. She was apt to gain trust not only because she "looked more like a local" but because she also could "seem more like them." Nurse Judd would often function as a preferred liaison, making a powerful difference in the health status of the Pohnpeian family because she was trusted, and therefore was able to change the way families viewed health issues.

When asked if that way of seeing and being was something Nanette knew versus something she was taught, she quickly responded: "It's the way I was brought up." In many ways, Nanette was brought up in a Hawaiian style, learning culture and values through storytelling. One profound story remembered and recounted many times was through the eyes of her mother during her registered nurse externship training in Missouri after she received her degree at St. Francis Hospital on O'ahu. The year was 1938. Nurse Beazley would catch the segregated bus—the norm in Missouri at the time—after working her shift at the local hospital. Crisply outfitted in her nurse whites and iconic headgear, she would accept the bus driver's request to sit up front. She would do so begrudgingly while enduring jeers and looks of disdain and bewilderment from both black and white patrons who passed her as they took their seats behind her: whites up front, blacks in the back, and Hawaiians at the discretion of the bus driver, apparently. Most times, she was given a privileged seat. Nanette's mother would recount these stories of racism to Nanette and her siblings. She would express how as an individual, being given advantage was a privilege that came with responsibility for those who had none.

Fast-forward one generation, to 1981, when Nanette's work at the John A. Burns School of Medicine began. While her training for it began as far back as childhood, she got there serendipitously in some ways. After her Peace Corps work and while still in Micronesia, Nanette did some collaborative work as a health manpower development liaison for JABSOM and the State of Hawai'i. This prompted a call from JABSOM dean of students, Dr. Benjamin Young, who was looking for a health-care provider with experience working with Pacific Islanders. He was ready to recruit for a federally funded grant program that was part of a manpower development project to include public health, nursing, and physician training needs. The mission of the program was to increase the number of underrepresented applicants, including ethnic minorities from Hawai'i and the Pacific Basin for professional health-care certifications.

"The opportunity spoke to me," Nanette explains. "I believed in the mission. And I believed in building the mission." Nanette recalls the early years as pioneering to say the least, and she often pounded the pavement looking for interested and qualified students from places like Hawai'i, American Sāmoa, Chuuk, Kosrae, Yap, Pohnpei, the Marshall Islands, Pālau, Saipan, and Guam. Her on-the-job education dealing with funding sources and advocating through policy and legislative action bloomed with the program's popularity and her own interest in making a difference. "In those days, affirmative action in education was synonymous with the training of the African American. We were carving from federal funding that seemed earmarked for that obvious need but we learned to pitch for the Pacific Islander and the Pacific Basin using both similar and unique premises." She credits much of her early success in understanding academic sustainability to the late senator Daniel Inouye. Through him and other respected John A. Burns School of Medicine mentors, she learned about the power of relationship building across divides to link academic, political, and grant agencies by using a shared language around Native Hawaiian systems building. Over her tenure, Nanette became skillful at federally funded grant work and strategically helped to move these monies to Hawai'i for the 'Imi Ho'ōla program. She learned much from the challenges of funding: how to use resources efficiently, how to collaborate, and how to prepare for every angle in order to get funding in the long run. To this day, Nanette's perseverance through bridge building is a working formula for 'Imi Ho'ōla.

When asked how she made her programmatic decisions or what she did when things got rough, her go-to answer was, "I always thought to myself, what would be the right thing to do for the students, and I would go that way." Nanette credits a long list of advisors and mentors who helped her navigate the waters of community engagement, legislative action, and academic achievement. She believed in the potential of all students, predicated on a foundation of giving back to the community where she grew up in and where she continues to live. Her longtime colleague and program-learning specialist, Karen Sakamoto says, "She has been a role model and inspiration to me. I strive daily to become a more culturally competent educator by opening my eyes to the needs and concerns of disadvantaged students and by making their dreams of becoming physicians a reality." Nanette Judd continues to be a formidable leader in the education of Native Hawaiians and other underrepresented students who have come through the 'Imi Ho'ōla program.

'Imi Ho'ōla Alumni Reflections

Patrice Ming-Lei Tim Sing, 'Imi Ho'ōla class of 1988–1989: Dr. Nanette Judd has been a mentor and trusted friend to me for more than twenty years. With each talk-story session we've shared, I've walked away refreshed, knowing she still continues to make a positive difference for all those around her, me included.

'Imi Ho'ōla was the lighthouse from which I sought advice and assurance of safe haven as I navigated through the difficult waters of my medical education. Dr. Judd was the ever-present lighthouse keeper, carefully tending the beam that still burns bright today.

Like other wonderful individuals in my circle of mentors, she and the program have taught me two important lessons.

First, choose medicine if it is *your* passion. 'Imi Ho'ōla can sharpen skills, but the heart for the profession and the work ethic it demands must come from inside you. The path to medicine has many forks, some which go down self-sabotaging dead ends. To a naive student lacking any experience in the life of medicine or the path through it, Nanette challenged me to identify those negative behaviors and gave me insight into choosing better ones. I spent just one year as a student of 'Imi Ho'ōla but I walked away with a lifetime of transformative insight into the daily practice of making choices toward my passion, medicine.

Second, my success in higher education, and ultimately medicine, was built on the shoulders of others before me. 'Imi Ho'ōla taught me about the kuleana (responsibility) to reach back with an extended arm and ready hand to help those in need behind me.

And that is why I am here, still learning medicine both as a faculty member of 'Imi Ho'ōla and a practicing physician, hoping our students will learn some of these same lessons . . . among other things, of course! Many thanks to those before me.

Leimomi Noel Kanagusuku, second-year medical student, 'Imi Ho'ōla class of 2013–2014: When I was a child, my grandmother always reminded me that "working hard will take you far," but I didn't realize what that meant exactly until I entered the 'Imi Ho'ōla Post-Baccalaureate Program. As the first in my family to go to college, I was groomed to do my best in school and to set my goals high, so naturally becoming a physician was one of those ambitions. I worked hard throughout high school and college, just like any other aspiring medical student, but I soon realized that public health was more of my passion. I focused less on the biological sciences and more on the social aspects of health, which led me to valuable experiences at the Hawai'i State Department of Health, and the Department of Native Hawaiian Health at JABSOM. However, when I received word that I had not been accepted into medical school at JABSOM, I felt that everything I'd worked for had been for nothing. They say everything happens for a reason, and though things had not gone exactly as planned, it was exactly what I needed; otherwise, I would not have been able to experience the 'Imi Ho'ōla program.

Much like a farmer tends to his crops as I used to do with my grandmother, this program has helped me blossom into what I am today. I was a dud seed, but the 'Imi Ho'ōla staff saw my potential and gave me a chance. By providing me with foundational biological sciences, the curriculum strengthened my knowledge base as well as my critical thinking skills. Perhaps my most academically challenging pursuit thus far, 'Imi nurtured my passion to work in underserved communities while testing my ability to truly learn, understand, and connect concepts. As I honed my scholastic prowess, I became more cognizant of my personal progress and ambitions. As a young Native Hawaiian, I knew that I wanted to help improve the health of my people but didn't know exactly how to pursue this. As an 'Imi Ho'ōla student, I discovered that one of my passions was teaching and I would be able to utilize these teaching skills to educate my future patients as a family medicine physician in my hometown of Wai'anae. I flourished in the environment 'Imi Ho'ōla provided, and after years of searching for a place to belong, I finally found my niche.

The 'Imi Ho'ōla program helped me to prepare for and enter medical school, but it did so much more than just providing me with an education. It instilled confidence and provided a new supportive 'ohana of classmates and program staff, an appreciation for my culture, and a revitalized passion for medicine. Most of all, 'Imi Ho'ōla has shown me how far a dream, hard work, and dedication will go with the right cultivation. I am proud and blessed to be part of the 'Imi Ho'ōla legacy, and I hope that I can give back to my people just as this program has done for me.

Akolea K. Ioane, 'Imi Ho'ōla class of 2009–2010: *Aia ma kahi hāiki* (it is in a narrow place) is said of an unborn infant. No plans are made until *puka nā maka i ke ao* (the eyes are seen in the daylight). This was one of many traditional concepts taught to me as a child, and like many other things, did not make sense until I was a parent myself.

I grew up in a small homestead community called Waikahalu'u on the Big Island of Hawai'i. There are no paved roads, no electricity, and no running water. This is where I watched my mother give birth to two of my siblings. As a ten-year-old, I watched as my sister was born on Easter day. I remember it distinctly. Before her birth, I had no idea that anything would change. I knew my mother was having a baby, but no one spoke about it and life went on as usual.

As my siblings and I passed by my parents' room, we heard the commotion and entered the room. My aunt explained to us what was going on. My siblings were uninterested, but I stayed. I was fascinated by the idea that a baby would enter the world through my mother.

Ka 'ōpu'u pua i mohala (a flower that begins to unfold) is said of a newborn infant. My father came bursting into the room the second he heard my sister's cry. His typically stern yet nonchalant demeanor melted away and emotions, which my father never expressed, appeared on his face. I was astonished by the attention he showered on the baby and my mother. My strict and rough father was cradling my sister as if she were a delicate flower, as though the breeze itself would bruise her face. At the age of seventeen I became pregnant. At eighteen, I became a single parent. When I saw my daughter for the first time, I was overwhelmed with affection for her. I then realized the true meaning of the Hawaiian proverbs that had never made much sense to me before. Only a parent can understand the loss of child and so to acknowledge an infant only after it is born is to protect you from the unbearable.

After high school, I pursued a career in nursing at the University of Hawai'i at Hilo. Following the completion of my degree, I began working at Bay Clinic, Inc., a community health center in Hilo. Nursing is difficult and requires a personality that exudes both confidence and competence. My nursing education not only provided me with lifelong friends, but helped me discover these valuable personality traits that are also required in medicine. The health-care providers at Bay Clinic recognized my potential for medicine, and they gave me responsibilities beyond that of a registered nurse. This made me see the limitations of my nursing license.

During my pregnancy, I formed an unexpected bond with my obstetrician, who encouraged me to pursue medicine. For four years, I worked as a full-time registered nurse and a part-time nurse researcher in addition to attending school at night to satisfy medical school prerequisites. Coming from a small-town university and a small Hawaiian community, I lacked guidance in my pursuit of medicine. By the time I took the Medical College Admission Test, I was burnt-out and exhausted. I wanted to achieve my dream so badly, but I just didn't have the resources. I wasn't prepared. Then I heard about 'Imi Ho'ōla from a friend who had completed the program. I applied and was accepted in 2009 and relocated to O'ahu. This was the first time that I had ever moved farther away than down the road from my family. I won't even attempt to describe the challenges I faced, especially the rigor and difficulty of the program. Most reading this won't have any experience to compare it with, and unless one is a participant in the program, it is impossible to conceive of what it entails.

Words can't express the influence and impact of ʻImi Hoʻōla on my life. Despite all that my daughter and I have had to sacrifice, ʻImi Hoʻōla provided me with the academic, professional and life skills required to complete medical school and be successful in the field of medicine. After completing the program, I entered the John A. Burns School of Medicine and graduated in 2014. I had a baby girl in my fourth year of medical school, got married during the summer after graduation, and I am now completing a residency in family medicine at Virginia Commonwealth University (VCU).

ʻO ka makapō wale nō ka mea hāpapa i ka pouli. If you have no direction in life, you will get nowhere, for the blind grope in the darkness. ʻImi Hoʻōla changed the trajectory of my life and allowed me to realize my dreams for my daughters and for myself. My daughters remain the positive force that drives me to continue to accomplish what might be difficult or even impossible. One of my greatest desires is to have them become aware of their maximum potential. I have realized that children often become what their communities and parents teach them to be. My daughters will only realize the infinite possibilities of their future if I guide and expose them to the possibilities. My oldest daughter fueled my desire to pursue medicine. Growing up in a tight-knit Hawaiian community taught me that we are responsible for our own families and surroundings. If we do not take responsibility for ourselves, we cannot expect anyone else to do so. My daughters have a mother who is a physician. My father has a daughter who is a physician, and my Hawaiian community has a member who is a physician. That is what the ʻImi Hoʻōla program has given to me.

Kelli-Ann Noelani Frank Voloch, ʻImi Hoʻōla class of 1993–1994: *Lawe i ka maʻalea a kūʻonoʻono* (acquire skill and make it deep). This proverbial saying begins my story in Makakilo on the island of Oʻahu, where I grew up as the oldest of three children. Fortunate to attend the Kamehameha Schools' Kapālama Campus at the bright age of four, my excitement for lifelong learning of science and Hawaiian culture emerged there. During the next few years, I faced several health challenges and multiple hospitalizations but soon became intrigued with medicine and the idea of becoming a physician. Despite high absenteeism, I was able to graduate from high school and begin my first year of college at Leeward Community College in the University of Hawaiʻi system. Although my dream was to travel to the mainland for college, it was placed on hold due to the financial burden of my medical bills and my parents' struggle to raise my siblings. Through perseverance, employment, and a generous financial aid package I was able to transfer to the College of Notre Dame in Belmont, California. I was blessed to have several mentors along with dedicated family and friends to guide me through the sophisticated milieu of college and medical school to become the first college graduate and physician in my family.

The ʻImi Hoʻōla Post-Baccalaureate Program provided me with an educational pathway toward a career in medicine and was my "dream builder." By serendipity, my medical school interviewer was Dr. Nanette Judd, who recognized my potential and encouraged me to apply to the program. This became one of the most incredible chapters of my life. The knowledge, skills, and confidence I developed in the program solidified my desire to pursue a career in medicine and allowed me to become the person I am today. It transformed my life by teaching me to embrace the chaos of life and remain steadfast in my goals and dreams. Following ʻImi Hoʻōla, I attended and graduated from medical school and went on to complete a pediatric residency in Honolulu at Kapiʻolani Medical Center for Women and Children. I now serve my community as a pediatrician and as an assistant professor in the ʻImi Hoʻōla program.

As a pediatrician at the Waiʻanae Coast Comprehensive Health Center, I have been honored to serve my ʻohana and patients over fifteen years, encouraging healthy eating and lifestyle choices in public and private schools, homes, and offices. I also have the privilege of mentoring and teaching in the ʻImi Hoʻōla program. It is an honor and dream come true for me to have the combination of an academic position and clinical practice. This dream has allowed me to advocate for our underserved and disadvantaged Native Hawaiian populations in rural areas of Hawaiʻi to improve their health and educational status. My patients, their families, and medical students consistently remind me about the intrigue and "art" of medicine and confirm my belief that dreams do come true. Thank you, Dr. Benjamin Young, Nanette Judd, and my ʻohana who all believed in me! To future *haumāna* (students), believe and you will achieve your dreams!

Summary

Since the program's inception in 1973, we have had 253 ʻImi alumni who have graduated from JABSOM. Many are now practicing in Hawaiʻi, Guam, U.S. Affiliated Pacific Islands (USAPI), American Sāmoa, and the continental United States. Thirty-three alumni are currently enrolled as medical students at JABSOM. The ʻImi Hoʻōla program is a very successful model for disadvantaged students to matriculate into, and graduate from, medical school. ʻImi Hoʻōla is a gift to the state of Hawaiʻi and continues to meet its goals of improving health care in Hawaiʻi and the Pacific Basin by increasing the number of primary care physicians serving those underserved areas and directly contributing to the diversity of the health-care workforce. ʻImi Hoʻōla is one of the most transformational and successful programs to improve health care in Hawai'i and the Pacific Basin. The dreams of many students from disadvantaged backgrounds were made possible by the program and its director for so many years, Dr. Nanette Judd. Dreams continue to be nurtured and made into a reality today under the auspicious leadership of current 'Imi Ho'ōla program director, Dr. Winona Mesiona Lee, and the generous funding support from The Queen's Health Systems.

The authors would like to acknowledge The Queen's Health Systems for their generous support of the 'Imi Ho'ōla Post-Baccalaureate Program. Funding for this program is made possible in part by The Queen's Health Systems Native Hawaiian Health Initiative. The views expressed in written materials or publications do not necessarily reflect the official policies of The Queen's Health Systems, nor does mention by trade names, commercial practices, or organizations imply endorsement by The Queen's Health Systems.

Kākou: Collaborative Cultural Competency

Martina Leialoha Kamaka, Vanessa S. Wong, Dee-Ann Carpenter, C. Malina Kaulukukui, and Gregory G. Maskarinec

Introduction

ʻAʻohe pau ka ʻike i ka hālau hoʻokahi.
All knowledge is not learned in one school[1]

Recognizing that medical education must prepare physicians to deal competently and compassionately with patients from all backgrounds, cultural competence must play an important role in health care. It is especially significant as it relates to eliminating the health disparities seen in different populations. The 2002 Institute of Medicine (IOM) Report, *Unequal Treatment*,[2] pointed out the physician factors, in addition to societal and social justice factors, that contribute to persistent health disparities.

In response to the IOM report, accreditation standards for medical schools now require that health disparities be addressed in the curriculum, cultural competency training be implemented and the social determinants of health be taught to all medical students.[3] At the University of Hawaiʻi at Mānoa John A. Burns School of Medicine (JABSOM), the Cultural Competency Curriculum (C3) Development Project within the Department of Native Hawaiian Health (DNHH) has taken the lead in creating innovative and sustainable cultural competency training initiatives for faculty, staff, and students at JABSOM. Although our efforts focus mainly on the disparities seen in the indigenous Native Hawaiian (NH) population, we believe that much of our training transcends ethnicity and is applicable across racial and cultural groups.

The interdisciplinary C3 team was formed in 2003 and is comprised of academic faculty and clinical faculty from different disciplines as well as community representatives. Current C3 efforts focus on integrating the expertise of its members into a comprehensive cultural competency curriculum addressing provider factors and training to reduce Native Hawaiian health disparities. Integral to these efforts is the understanding that health and wellness for Native Hawaiians must be holistic in nature. Health must include the balance of body, mind, and spirit as well as a balance between the individual/family/community, the environment, and God/higher pow-

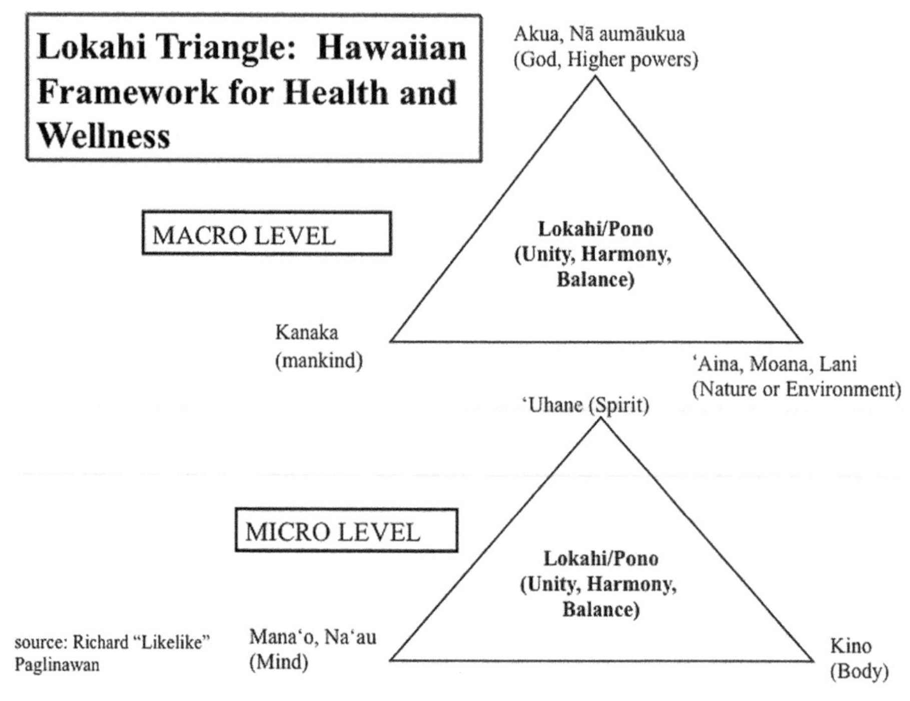

Figure 6.1. Lōkahi Triangle by M. Kamaka.

ers. The diagrams above illustrate this holistic Native Hawaiian worldview (see Figure 6.1).[4] Health disparities then, in the Native Hawaiian framework, are a result of the imbalances present in the life of a person, as well as that in a person's family and community. The source or cause of the imbalances may vary, but everything is interrelated. What affects one thing, will affect the rest.

"Culture" or cultural competency is difficult to teach in the classroom. Therefore, the C3 project team utilizes a variety of different teaching methodologies to make the topic interesting and relevant. Methodologies include lecture, small group discussion, problem-based learning, demonstration, role-play, standardized patient experiences, and experiential learning such as cultural immersion. Community partners and cultural practitioners are instrumental in the delivery of each of these methodologies. This reiterates a critical guiding principle for the C3 project, which comes from a Native Hawaiian proverbial saying or 'ōlelo no'eau, "*'a'ohe pau ka 'ike i ka hālau ho'okahi*" (all knowledge is not learned in one school).[5] This chapter examines the history of these efforts and discusses several initiatives including cultural immersion, a series of workshops, standardized patient exercises, modifications to JABSOM's problem-based-learning (PBL) curriculum and electives in Native Hawaiian health.

The Creation of C3

E hana mua a pa'a ke kahua mamua o ka a'o ana aku ia ha'i.
Build yourself a firm foundation before teaching others[6]

Cultural competency, as described by the U.S. Department of Health and Human Services is "a set of congruent behaviors, knowledge, attitudes, and policies that come together in a system, organization, or among professionals that enables effective work in cross-cultural situations."[7] The late 1990s in Hawai'i saw several movements, both community and university based, to address cultural competency and Native Hawaiian health disparities. Community initiatives included the 1998 Ka 'Uhane Lōkahi–Native Hawaiian health and wellness summit and the 1999 statewide NHLBI (National Heart, Lung, Blood Institute) cardiovascular education programs. These two efforts created the first opportunities for Native Hawaiian physicians to network and strategize around the topic of Native Hawaiian health disparities. Critical to this was the realization among the physicians that they needed cultural training and grounding themselves. In response to these concerns, the 'Ahahui o nā Kauka (Association of Native Hawaiian Physicians) was established.

In the meantime, cultural competency training efforts began at JABSOM in the late 1990s under the direction of Dr. Benjamin Young, the director for the HRSA (Health Resources and Services Administration)–funded Native Hawaiian Center of Excellence (NHCOE). Dr. Young quickly recognized that most JABSOM faculty lacked an awareness of Native Hawaiian health disparities. Faculty-oriented workshops were designed to increase awareness of Native Hawaiian health issues, target cultural competency training, and introduce faculty to NH traditional healers and concepts regarding wellness. In addition, the NHCOE also understood that a multidisciplinary team would best address Native Hawaiian culture and cultural competency. In 2003, each department of the medical school was invited to designate one faculty member to join the effort. Expertise outside of the medical school was sought as well. The team came to be called the Cultural Competency Curriculum Development team or C3.

Initial C3 members included faculty from the Departments of Native Hawaiian Health, Psychiatry, Family Medicine, and Internal Medicine as well as the School of Social Work and the Hawai'i State Department of Health. Since its inception, the team has expanded to include members from the Office of Medical Education, the Department of Surgery, community physicians, and members of community organizations such as Queen's Hospital. Members' expertise includes medicine, social work, public health, business, and cultural anthropology, as well as NH cultural practices. The C3 team is also fortunate to benefit from the guidance of prominent Native Hawaiian health advocates such as Richard Kekuni Blaisdell, MD, and Claire Hughes, DrPH, RD.

The NHCOE sponsored several workshops over five years, the most significant a novel cultural competency curriculum developed in the spring of 2000 for physicians by the NHCOE, the 'Ahahui o nā Kauka, and the Protect Kaho'olawe 'Ohana (PKO). Physician participants took part in an intense cultural immersion experience (designed by the PKO) coupled with a medical CME (continuing medical education) program. The curriculum was delivered on the island of Kaho'olawe, a land rich in cultural resources but long a target of military bombing and destructive introduced animal ranching and grazing. The goal was to bridge the gap between the Western training of the physicians and traditional approaches to health and healing, while having the Island of Kaho'olawe serve as a vivid metaphor of NH trauma and current efforts at renewal and healing.

The conference proved to be deeply moving and inspirational for the participants.[8] "Learning occurred on many levels"[9] and for many, a personal transformation happened that facilitated a "connectedness" to land and ancestors. Generational responsibility, cultural pride, and increased awareness of spirituality were cultivated. At a follow-up focus group session, as many as 50 percent of those present felt that the experience had improved their communication with patients as well as increased their openness to traditional healing and awareness of cultural conflicts.[10] With the formation of the Department of Native Hawaiian Health in 2003, cultural competency training for medical students was added as a key area of focus for the department and the C3 project was integrated into the department along with the NHCOE and the 'Imi Ho'ola post-baccalaureate program.

As cultural competency training was a relatively new, rapidly developing field in medical schools, there was no consensus on how to teach it. The C3 team realized that Native Hawaiian culture had to be the curriculum's foundation. As culture is difficult to teach in a didactic format, the C3 team decided early on that it would be necessary to utilize a variety of different teaching methodologies. In addition, existing JABSOM curricula were modified as needed and new curricular components were introduced. Furthermore, many hours were spent debating the appropriateness of the term "cultural competency." The C3 team recognized that no one can truly be competent in another's culture. Many newer and better terms currently exist in this field such as cultural humility, cultural safety, cultural resonance, and cultural responsiveness. However, we continue to use "cultural competency" as it is the term used by the federal funders for the C3 project. Nevertheless, we were determined to keep the curriculum rooted in Native Hawaiian values.[11] Key Hawaiian values taught in our curriculum include *aloha* (to care for, love);

mālama (to take care of); *'imi 'ike* (to seek knowledge); *lokomaika'i* (to share); *olakino maika'i* (to be healthy); and *kōkua aku, kōkua mai* (reciprocity). The emphasis on reviewing and incorporating parts of past and current cultural competency efforts, building a multidisciplinary team, deciding on which teaching methodologies to use and rooting all of it in Hawaiian culture provided the team with a strong foundation from which to begin its teaching efforts.

The Relationship between Cultural Historical Trauma and Health Disparities

Medical students cannot be expected to understand or know how to address Native Hawaiian health disparities without understanding its causes. Early in the first year, students learn about Hawaiian history, especially as it relates to the impact of colonization, including loss of sovereignty, land, culture, societal norms, and even family. These factors combined with the devastating population decline (88–95 percent, depending on population estimates in 1778) due to introduction of foreign disease,[12] result in a phenomenon known as cultural, historical, or intergenerational trauma.[13]

These losses result in chronic cumulative emotional and psychological wounding and unresolved grief that can be carried across generations. This phenomenon can be found in colonized indigenous peoples across the world, where it appears in communal feelings of family and social disruptions, regular re-experiencing of the trauma via racism and negative stereotyping, and lack of resolution of the communal pain with chronic existential grief manifested in destructive behaviors such as addictions and family violence.[14,15,16,17]

The knowledge about the long-range negative consequences of cumulative trauma was enhanced by an extensive study by the Center of Disease Control and Kaiser Permanente of approximately 17,000 Kaiser patients in the 1990s. The results showed a powerful relationship between our emotional experiences as children and their negative effects on our physical and mental health as adults. If the trauma issues are not addressed and/or if there is an absence of protective factors in the child's life, these negative experiences play major causal roles in chronic disease and adult mortality.[18] Known as the Adverse Childhood Experiences Study (ACE), researchers paired contemporary findings about brain research with the epidemiology of the ACE study, and revealed how trauma creates neurobiological deficits in children affecting every facet of their lives over their life span.[19]

Trauma impacts not only individuals across life spans but also communities across generations. Specifically, Hawai'i's modern post–Western contact history is characterized by swift and multiple changes within Hawaiian culture and society during the late eighteenth and nineteenth centuries. These changes began with the arrival of Captain James Cook in 1778, followed by foreign traders, who brought Western technologies, social norms, religion, capitalism, and politics to the islands, along with infectious diseases for which Hawaiians had no immunity. Exposure to Western culture, its norms and religion, led to critical changes such as the removal of certain gender and social prohibitions by the ruling chiefs in 1819. Without the traditional spiritual and social practices that defined how people interacted with each other, their environment, and their gods, an overwhelming void was created leading to confusion and loss for large segments of the population.[20]

Interestingly, the arrival of Calvinist missionaries from the United States in 1820 came at a time when Hawaiians were reeling from these losses, and Christianity filled that void. However, it came with a cultural price of forced assimilation into a Western worldview. Nevertheless, the catastrophic event that most disrupted the well-being of Hawaiians was the overthrow of the Hawaiian monarchy in 1893, an event that still reverberates in the spirits of contemporary Hawaiians. The legacy of colonization for Native Hawaiians includes racism, low socioeconomic status, and loss of sovereignty, language, land, and cultural and spiritual practices, including traditional healing practices, resulting ultimately in current Native Hawaiian health disparities.

However, as ensuing generations move further away from the major precipitating traumatic events that happened in Hawai'i, some communities have demonstrated a capacity for resiliency and effective leadership in advancing initiatives that restore traditional cultural practices and cultural pride, and are enjoying economic, educational, and political successes.[21] Yet, far too many health practitioners are still faced with patients who are affected by "injury where blood doesn't flow."[22] Common themes presented by patients may be passivity about their own health needs, continued self-destructive behaviors, and distrust of health-care professionals. This reinforces the importance of training health-care professionals who are well practiced in the principles of cultural humility and culturally competent care. Health-care providers must be able to engage not only the patient, but also the family and the broader community in the collaborative partnering needed for effective treatment.

Cultural Immersion

Ma ka hana ka 'ike[23]
In doing, one learns

Initial C3 efforts were guided by the results of a series of focus groups in 2004 targeting Native Hawaiian patients, physicians, and students. The physicians were recruited from the group of Kaho'olawe participants. In that study, two primary themes emerged: cultural competency must be included in physician training, and the role of traditional healing must be addressed. These themes, along with a strong physician recommendation for time devoted to self-awareness and experiential learning, guided our initial curricular efforts.[24] Building on the experience of the Kaho'olawe physician cultural immersion program, the C3 team developed the Native Hawaiian cultural immersion weekend for first-year medical students in 2006.

The three-day Native Hawaiian cultural immersion is a unique, strengths-based, experiential learning experience designed to enhance quality medical care for the underserved and to address persistent health disparities in our state. Evaluation by pre- and post-testing has shown that our students, whether or not they are from Hawai'i, have much to learn about Native Hawaiian patients, their varied cultures, social history, and attitudes toward health care, as well as their own future medical practices. Our experiential curriculum promotes learning through "active" participation ("doing"—touching, feeling, on an emotional and spiritual level) as well as introduces students to the social determinants of health and principles of social justice. The immersion experience aims to provide students with insights and skills to improve their interactions with Native Hawaiian patients as well as those from other underserved populations. By "living" in a culture, even if only for three days, seeing, hearing, and experiencing its problems and its successes, resiliencies, and challenges in a real-life setting, a foundation is being set for acquiring attitudes, knowledge, and skills that are reinforced through our didactic curriculum.

The immersion weekend is linked to a medical school problem-based-learning case wherein the students learn about Native Hawaiian health disparities. The weekend takes place on the rural Wai'anae Coast of O'ahu Island in a community that is predominantly Native Hawaiian. Students are randomly selected due to curricular time, space, and budget constraints. We are able to take up to 25 percent of the first-year class. Preparation for this type of experience is critical; students spend time familiarizing themselves with Native Hawaiian values and traditional healing practices as well as learning the cultural protocols that will be used throughout the weekend.

During the weekend, lessons and experiences center upon the Hawaiian worldview of health and wellness.[25] Intellectual growth occurs around learning about traditional healing, navigation, agriculture, and water management practices as well as types of patient-physician communication styles appropriate for our patients. Understanding one's own genealogy and sense of place encourages emotional and mental growth. These are some of the tools students use to aid in the identification of their own values, assumptions, and biases that may serve to support and/or thwart effective patient care. Physical nurturing occurs through engaging in traditional food preparation, service learning, and physical activities specific to Hawaiian culture. Community needs are addressed through understanding the sense of place that incorporates history, community resources, and challenges such as conflicts over land, water, and sovereignty—all in the context of social justice. Spirituality comes into play through the engagement in traditional protocols and acknowledgment of the Native Hawaiian spiritual connection to 'āina.

Throughout the weekend, the significance of land-based spirituality and individual and community kuleana for caring for our home and its people are continually reinforced. The faculty attempt to bridge all of the different events and experiences to tie in to the whole concept of using the strengths of a culture as well as community resources to help care for patients, particularly our Native Hawaiian patients, where effective treatment might be one that incorporates a return to traditional practices that nourish not only the body but also the mind and the soul.

Native Hawaiian Health Elective for First-Year Students

Cultural activities engage students, faculty, and staff with the intent of encouraging increased self-awareness, respect for diversity of cultures, and the importance of traditional cultural beliefs in the health and well-being of patients and their families. Cultural competency and cultural humility require community input, and therefore teaching must occur beyond the walls of the traditional classroom.

JABSOM requires that first-year medical students spend four hours per week in a yearlong community health elective of their choosing to develop an appreciation of the role of the community in their patients' health. One elective that is available to the students as part of the C3 curriculum is *Native Hawaiian Health: Past, Present, Future.* This multidimensional course exposes students to Native Hawaiian health across a continuum, spanning pre–Western contact to the present day. This course has been modified over the years;[26] in its current and longest-lasting form, it utilizes a combination of didactics, hands-on workshops, and field trips to help students gain a better understanding of the holistic nature of Native Hawaiian health and health-care practices. Service-learning projects are interwoven throughout the course, connecting the *past* with the *present* and looking toward the *future.*

Native Hawaiian Health: Past introduces students to traditional healing practices and the importance of the Native Hawaiian relationship to the land and environmental resources, with respect to health. The elective stresses the critical role of the healthy *ahupua'a* (mountain to sea land division). Students learn protocol, work closely with traditional healers, and engage in service-learning opportunities that promote an understanding of the relationship between healthy 'aina, kuleana, and health.

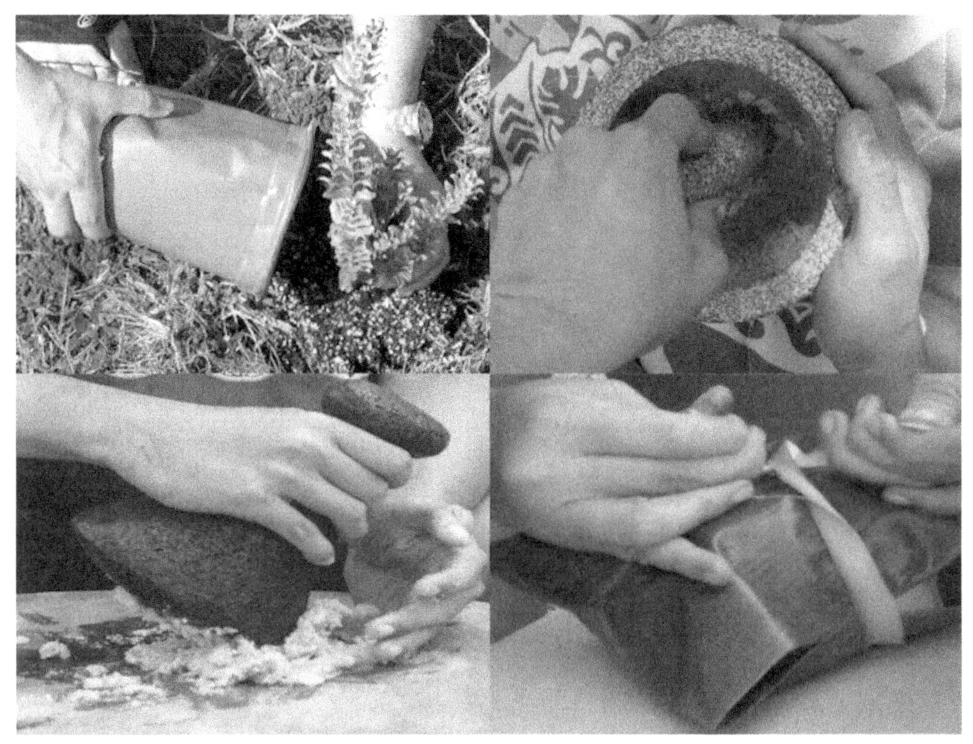

Figure 6.2. “Hands” collage by Leslie Yap is an example of experiential learning. Image courtesy of M. Kamaka.

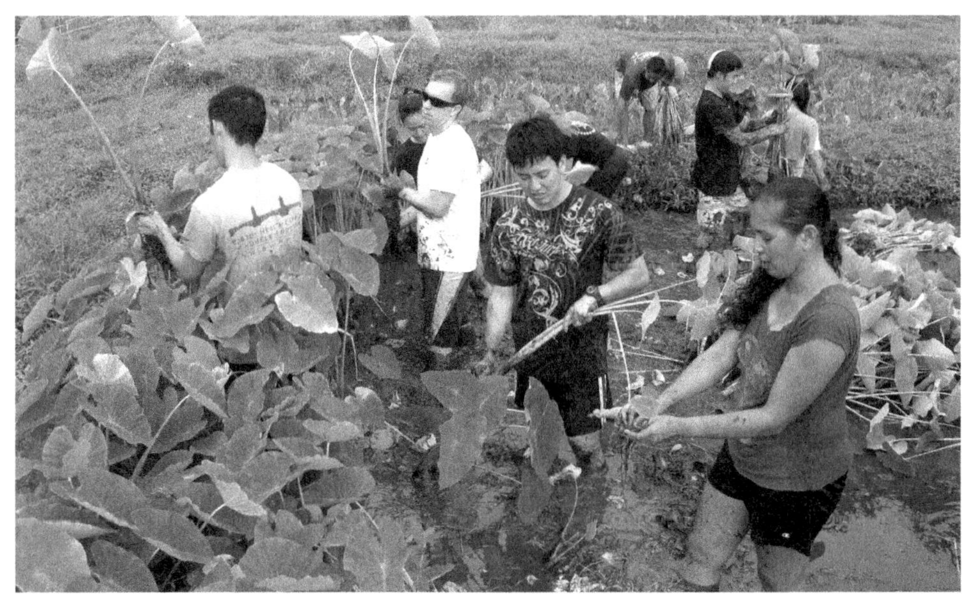

Figure 6.3. Students and faculty in *lo‘i kalo* (taro patch) at Papahana Kuaola by Leslie Yap. Image courtesy of photographer.

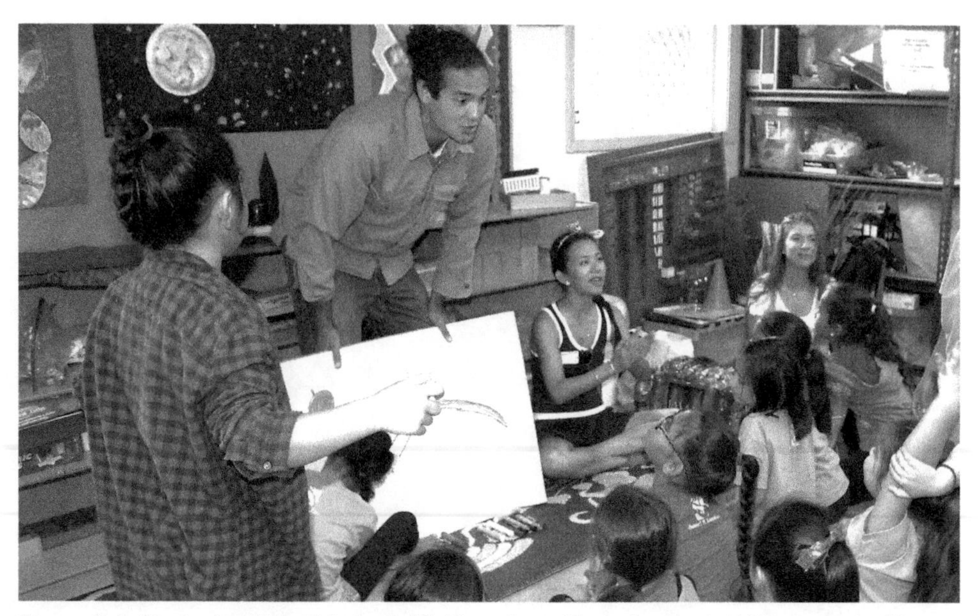

Figure 6.4. Students at Ke Kula ʻo S. M. Kamakau. Photo by Nash Witten, used with permission.

Native Hawaiian Health: Present examines the current status of Native Hawaiian health, including health disparities. Additional activities in this section include research into current newsworthy topics impacting the Native Hawaiian community ranging from cultural practices to civilian and military uses of important agricultural and sacred lands. Finally students learn about current efforts and community resources targeting healthy people, communities, and lifestyles. They have the opportunity to get involved in these projects and develop relationships with communities and organizations to which they can then refer their patients and families.

Native Hawaiian Health: Future explores current research being conducted in Native Hawaiian communities to address health disparities. Students consider the findings of these projects and the potential for significant impact on the overall health outcomes of the Native Hawaiian community. At the end of the year, students participate in a one-and-a-half-day "mini-immersion" modeled after the longer weekend immersion previously described. In addition, students are asked to reflect on how the lessons of this course will affect their future practices. As faculty, we believe that a critical lesson for students is the significance of differing perspectives of "healing" for patients. The Western allopathic goal of "curing" is, by definition, biological and individualistic. "Healing" takes a patient on a subjective and personal journey. "Indigenous healing" is defined as a spiritual process that includes a necessary change and cultural renewal.[27] Indigenous healing tends to be an interrelated phenomenon and focuses on the connections between family, community, culture, and nature, particularly relative to the ʻāina. This is the overarching concept that we hope our students understand at the end of the course.

Colloquia: The Interaction of Culture and Medicine

Soon after the immersion experiences began, the C3 team was offered some community health colloquia time to enable a cultural competency curriculum to reach all first-year medical students. Community health colloquia are offered for four hours every quarter. Over the past six years, the C3 cultural competency curricular efforts have expanded to three of the four colloquia, in addition to an "Introduction to Native Hawaiian Health" lecture offered in the first block of medical school. As much as possible, colloquia are timed to cover relevant material that correlates with other course material being offered at the medical school. The colloquia are titled "The Interaction of Culture and Medicine." Students learn about cultural competency, the traditional NH concepts around health and wellness, health disparities, and cultural trauma. Demonstrations and seminars by traditional healers are highlights of the workshops. By exposing the students to traditional healers early in their training, we hope to break down barriers between the two medical practices and facilitate discussion that students may have in the future with healers as they care for mutual patients.

During the colloquia, the students also participate in small group sessions that utilize genealogy and sense of place as tools to stimulate self-awareness. In addition, we teach the Four Habits Model[28] of patient engagement followed by a role-play exercise where each student has an opportunity to interview a patient and practice these skills. Our final colloquium is linked to a standardized patient experience that likewise is linked to a PBL case the students are studying. During that time, we review the student assessments of the standardized patient encounters, as well as feature a Native Hawaiian patient panel and a rural health panel.

Standardized Patients and PBL

We have worked to integrate a longitudinal patient scenario for students in their first and second years of medical school extending over three problem-based learning (PBL) cases and a cross-cultural standardized patient (SP) exercise, built around the experiences of a Native Hawaiian patient, "Robert Kealoha," whom the students first meet early in the curriculum when he is newly diagnosed with type 2 diabetes mellitus. They meet him again in subsequent "units" as he ages and develops complications. As part of the third unit, students have an SP session with Mr. Kealoha and his wife. The design of the SP examination approximates an actual patient encounter but focuses on history taking, and students are tasked with uncovering cultural issues. Also, key teaching points are drawn on the "Four Habits" model students learn in an earlier colloquium. The SP encounter is videotaped and reviewed by faculty preceptors, who choose key moments for teaching clips that are shared with the students along with a triangulated assessment completed by the preceptors, the "patients," and the students. In addition, we recently added Mr. Kealoha as a simulation lab case for the transition unit before third-year clerkships. We collaborate with the Office of Medical Education and the Department of Geriatrics to integrate multiple issues including patient-physician communication, cultural sensitivity, and interdisciplinary team care.

Native Hawaiian Health Elective for Fourth-Year Students

For the past decade, the medical school has offered a four-week elective for senior JABSOM and visiting students who are interested in exploring more about the role of and possible interaction between traditional healing practices and Western medicine in Native Hawaiian populations. Typically, students do some clinical work with an NH physician or a physician who works in an NH community, and spend time with a traditional healer, in addition to doing community service work and independent study.

A sample elective experience on O'ahu would include an orientation period learning about NH history and culture, working with a Native Hawaiian primary care practitioner in a medical clinic, and performing community service with Na Lomilomi o Papakolea once a week by providing health screenings and blood pressure reading for community members visiting lomilomi (traditional Hawaiian body work) practitioners.[29] These traditional healers then provide shadowing experiences. If the student chooses to do the elective on a neighbor island, similar experiences are arranged depending on the resources and practitioners available.

Challenges and Future Directions

'A'ohe hana nui ke alu 'ia[30]
No task is too big when done together by all

One of the biggest challenges for C3 has been evaluation of our programs. Although the assessment of cultural competency efforts is challenging, the DNHH C3 project has found that qualitative student reflections can be the most useful for gauging meaningful impact on students. Nevertheless, we understood that we needed to add quantitative information to student reflections to more completely demonstrate impact to funders and administrators. We found it helpful to utilize preexisting quantitative tools and adapt them for our needs. For the immersion, we used a non-medical education assessment tool and modified it with the help of one of the original authors. For the standardized patient assessment tool, we used one originally developed by the Department of Family Medicine, then adapted by the Department of Surgery, and finally modified slightly by the C3 project.

Other challenges for the cultural competency curriculum include financial support and time. Finding more curricular time in a very busy medical education schedule is challenging and time commitments for faculty can be intense, especially considering many of the activities occur on weekends. Ideally, we would like to incorporate some of the topics covered in the elective and immersion into the curriculum for *all* of the students to experience. Budget is always an issue. We have been fortunate to have the immersion institutionalized and federal grant support through the NHCOE. Nevertheless, C3 needs to look toward long-term sustainability as we continue plans to expand cultural sensitivity training at JABSOM.

Conclusions

He pūko'a kani 'āina[31]
A coral reef grows into an island

We believe our curriculum goes beyond "cultural competency," which tends to focus primarily on the traditional cultural concepts and practices of patients and their communities. We advocate for "cultural humility" as a goal in multicultural physician education.[32] Cultural humility includes the practitioner's lifelong commitment to self-reflection and self-evaluation, to equalizing the inherent power imbalance in patient-physician dynamics, and to developing non-paternalistic partnerships with their communities in the service of community well-being.

While our project addresses specific cultural concerns of our local setting and its host culture, we suggest that similarly designed curricular interventions such as local immersions, courses, and culturally standardized patients concentrating on one culture whose members typically face health disparities would assist other schools in improving the cultural humility of their students, resulting in more sensitive caring for all patients.

Health is a state of complete physical, mental, and social well-being, not merely the absence of disease or infirmity. In our Hawaiian context, that includes not only our own health, but that of our 'ohana, our community, and

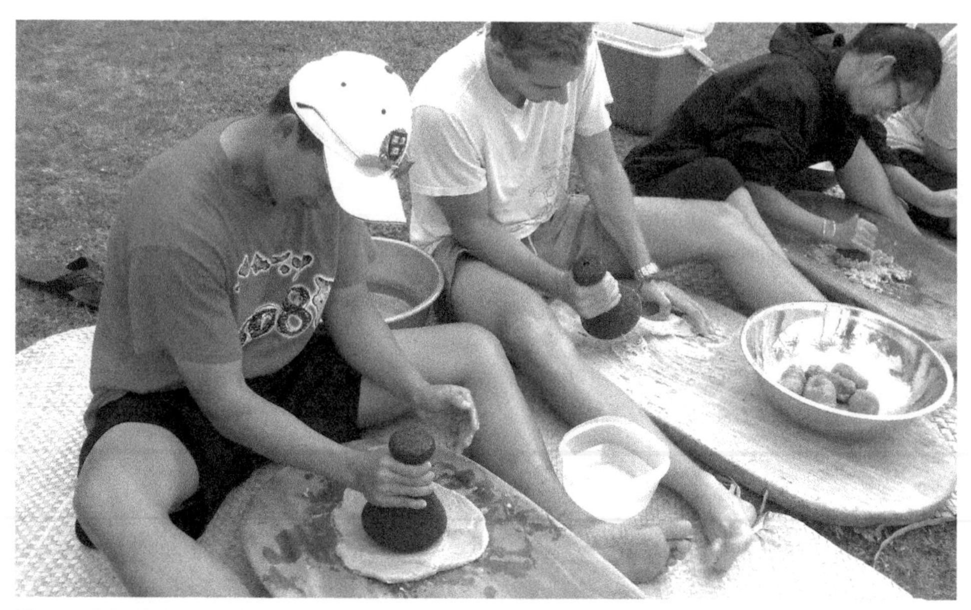
Figure 5.5. Making *pa'i'ai* (pounded steamed taro root) in Punalu'u. Photo by Nash Witten, used with permission.

our land and environment. In addition, we need to train physicians to recognize that health is a fundamental human right and that gross inequalities in health care are politically, socially, and economically unacceptable.[33] To do so, we must address culture; as a recent *Lancet* cover article states: "The systematic neglect of culture in health is the single biggest barrier to advancement of the highest attainable standard of health worldwide (availability, accessibility, acceptability, and quality)."[34] As Rudolph Virchow observed, "Do we not always find the diseases of the populace traceable to defects in society?"[35] Addressing culture in medical education is one more step toward correcting society's defects. This is not always easily done. There can be resistance, both outright and subtle, toward what might be considered "low-yield" information that will not be included in exams and "soft science" (social sciences, behavioral sciences), from not only students but institutions themselves.

Nevertheless, it has been our experience that the JABSOM cultural competency curriculum has proven its worth. Our efforts are well received by faculty and students and we have been able to build on our small initial efforts and grow, integrating ourselves more into the overall curriculum. Community engagement and consultation, collaboration with other faculty, and consideration for where our efforts fit best within JABSOM's medical curriculum are critical features for our current and future efforts. It's been exciting to be a part of this work and watch our small curricular "coral reef" grow into an "island" that will continue to expand and help nurture future physicians.

The authors would like to acknowledge the following for the financial support of our programs: JABSOM DNHH and Native Hawaiian Center of Excellence (HRSA grant 2D34HP16044), JABSOM Office of Medical Education, University of Hawai'i SEED grant, University of Hawai'i at Mānoa Kuali'i Council, and the JABSOM Dean's Office. *Mahalo* (thank you) to all of our many community partners, some of whom include 'Ai Pōhaku, Ānuenue Canoe Club, Board of Water Supply, Cultural Center at Ka'ala, Ho'oulu 'Āina, Ka Mō'ī Canoe Club, Kamehameha Schools, Kānehunamoku, Ke Kula o Kamakau, Keānuenue Farms and 'Ohana Bishop, Mālama Makua, Paepae o He'eia, Papa Ola Lōkahi, Papahana Kuaola, Polynesian Voyaging Society, Wahiawa Hawaiian Civic Club (Kūkaniloko), Wa'ianae Coast Comprehensive Health Center, and many other individual volunteers, UH faculty, and traditional healers. We are honored to have you as part of our teaching team. Finally, this chapter is dedicated to the memory of Richard "Likeke" Paglinawan, MSW, 'Ōlohe Lua. We are very grateful for his support and advice and for the wisdom that he shared with us and our students since our program's inception.

NOTES

1. Mary Kawena Pukui, *'Ōlelo No'eau: Hawaiian Proverbs and Poetical Sayings* (Honolulu: Bishop Museum Press, 1983), 24.
2. Brian Smedley, *Unequal Treatment: Confronting Racial and Ethnic Disparities in Health Care* (Washington, DC: Institute of Medicine of the National Academy Press, 2002).
3. *Functions and Structure of a Medical School: Standards for Accreditation of Medical Education Programs Leading to the M.D. Degree,* LCME (Liaison Committee on Medical Education, 2015), accessed on October 8, 2015, http://www.lcme.org/publications.htm, accessed October 8, 2015.
4. Richard Paglinawan, "Ho'oponopono" (Lecture at the John A. Burns School of Medicine, September 1, 2009).
5. Pukui, *'Ōlelo No'eau,* 24.
6. Ibid., 34.
7. U.S. Department of Health and Human Services Office of Minority Health, *Assuring Cultural Competence in Health Care: Recommendations for National Standards and Outcomes-Focused Research Agenda* (Washington, DC: U.S. Government Printing Office, 2000).
8. Martina Kamaka and N. Emmett Aluli, "Utilizing Cultural Immersion in a Cultural Competency Curriculum: A Conference Report," *Pacific Health Dialog* 8 (2001): 423–428.
9. Martina Kamaka, "Cultural Immersion in a Cultural Competency Curriculum," *Academic Medicine* 76 (2001): 512.
10. Martina Kamaka, "Designing a Cultural Competency Curriculum: Asking the Stakeholders," *Hawaii Medical Journal* 69, Suppl. 3 (2010): 31–34.
11. Dee-Ann Carpenter, Martina Kamaka, and C. Malina Kaulukukui, "An Innovative Approach to Developing a Cultural Competency Curriculum; Efforts at the John

A. Burns School of Medicine, Department of Native Hawaiian Health," *Hawaii Medical Journal* 70, Suppl. 2 (2011): 15–19.

12. Ian Anderson et al., "Indigenous Health in Australia, New Zealand, and the Pacific," *The Lancet* 367 (2006): 1775–1785.

13. Maria Braveheart and Lemyra DeBruyn, "The American Indian Holocaust: Healing Historical Unresolved Grief," *American Indian and Alaska Native Mental Health Research: Journal of the National Center* 8 (1998): 60–82.

14. Michelle Sotero, "A Conceptual Model of Historical Trauma: Implications for Public Health Practice and Research," *Journal of Health Disparities Research and Practice* 1 (2006): 93–108.

15. Elizabeth Fast and Delphine Collin-Vezina, "Historical Trauma, Race-based Trauma and Resilience of Indigenous Peoples: A Literature Review," *First Peoples Review* 5 (2010): 126–136.

16. "Bringing Them Home: The 'Stolen Children' Report (1997)," Australian Human Rights Commission, https://www.humanrights.gov.au/our-work/aboriginal-and-torres-strait-islander-social-justice/publications/bringing-them-home-stolen, accessed June 1, 2015.

17. Eduardo Duran, *Healing the Soul Wound: Counseling with American Indians and other Native Peoples* (New York: Teachers College Press, 2006).

18. Vincent Felitti et al., "Relationship of Childhood Abuse and Household Dysfunction to Many of the Leading Causes of Death in Adults: The Adverse Childhood Experiences (ACE) Study," *American Journal of Preventive Medicine* 14 (1998): 245–258.

19. Robert Anda et al., "The Enduring Effects of Abuse and Related Experiences in Childhood: A Convergence of Evidence from Neurobiology and Epidemiology," *European Archive of Psychiatry and Clinical Neuroscience* 256 (2006): 174–186.

20. Bud Cook, Kelly Withy, and Lucia Tarallo-Jensen, "Cultural Trauma, Hawaiian Spirituality, and Contemporary Health Status," *Californian Journal of Health Promotion, Special Issue: Hawaii* 1 (2003): 10–24.

21. Kai Duponte et al., "'Ike Hawai'i—A Training Program for Working with Native Hawaiians," *Journal of Indigenous Voices in Social Work* 1 (2010): 1–24.

22. Evelyn Einhaeuser, "Eduardo Duran: Healing the Soul Wound," *Synergies in Healing Journal* (2015), http://www.synergies-journal.com/synergies/2015/4/2/eduardo-duran-overcoming-historical-trauma, accessed May 31, 2015.

23. Pukui, *'Ōlelo No'eau*, 227.

24. Martina Kamaka, Diane Paloma, and Gregory Maskarinec, "Recommendations for Medical Training: A Native Hawaiian Patient Perspective," *Hawaii Medical Journal* 71, Suppl. (2011): 31–34.

25. Paglinawan, "Ho'oponopono."

26. Martina Kamaka, "Native Hawaiian Health Past, Present, Future: The Genesis of a Course," in *Leaders in Indigenous Medical Education Network 2013, LIME Good Practice Case Studies*, vol. 2 (Melbourne: Onemda VicHealth Koori Health Unit, University of Melbourne, 2013), 5–9.

27. Gregory Phillips, *Addictions and Healing in Aboriginal Country* (Canberrra: Aboriginal Studies Press, 2003), 1–210.

28. Terry Stein, Ed Krupat, and Richard Frankel, "Talking with Patients. Using the Four Habits Model," The Permanente Medical Group Physician Education and Development, 2011, http://kpsaccme.com/CME/PPI/PPI_Handout1_Stein_17.pdf, accessed October 9, 2015.

29. Adrienne Dillard et al., "Case Report from the Field: Integrating Hawaiian and Western Healing Arts in Papakōlea," *Hawaii Journal of Medicine & Public Health* 73, Suppl. 3 (2014): 26–28.

30. Pukui, *'Ōlelo No'eau*, 18.

31. Ibid., 100.

32. Melanie Tervalon and Jann Murray-Garcia, "Cultural Humility versus Cultural Competence: A Critical Distinction in Defining Physician Training Outcomes in Multicultural Education," *Journal of Healthcare for the Poor and Underserved* 9 (1998): 117–125.

33. Allen Hixon and Gregory Maskarinec, "The Declaration of Alma Ata on its Thirtieth Anniversary: Its Relevance for Family Medicine Today," *Family Medicine* 40 (2008): 584–587.

34. David Napier et al., "Culture and Health," *The Lancet* 384 (2014): 1607–1639.

35. Allen Hixon et al., "Social Justice: The Heart of Medical Education," *Social Medicine* 7 (2013): 153–160.

BIBLIOGRAPHY

Anda, Robert, Vincent Felitti, J. Douglas Bremner, John Walker, Charles Whitfield, Bruce Perry, Shante Dube, and Wayne Giles. "The Enduring Effects of Abuse and Related Adverse Experiences in Childhood." *European Archives of Psychiatry and Clinical Neuroscience* 256 (2005): 174–186.

Anderson, Ian, Sue Crengle, Martina Kamaka, Tai-Ho Chen, Neal Palafox, and Lisa Jackson-Pulver. "Indigenous Health in Australia, New Zealand, and the Pacific." *The Lancet* 367 (2006): 1775–1785.

Australian Human Rights Commission. "Bringing Them Home: The 'Stolen Children' Report (1997)." https://www.humanrights.gov.au/our-work/aboriginal-and-torres-strait-islander-social-justice/publications/bringing-them-home-stolen. Accessed June 1, 2015.

Braveheart, Maria, and Lemyra DeBruyn. "The American Indian Holocaust: Healing Historical Unresolved Grief." *American Indian and Alaska Native Mental Health Research (AIANMHR)* 8 (1998): 60–82.

Carpenter, Dee-Ann, Martina Kamaka, and C. Malina Kaulukukui. "An Innovative Approach to Developing a Cultural Competency Curriculum Efforts at the John A. Burns School of Medicine, Department of Native Hawaiian Health." *Hawaii Medical Journal* 70, Suppl. 2 (2011): 15–19.

Cook, Bud, Kelley Withy, and Lucia Jensen. "Cultural Trauma, Hawaiian Spirituality, and Contemporary Health Status." *Californian Journal of Health Promotion, Special Issue: Hawaii* 1 (2003): 10–24.

Dillard, Adrienne, Dee-Ann Carpenter, Ethel Mau, and B. Puni Kekauoha. "Case Report from the Field: Integrating Hawaiian and Western Healing Arts in Papakōlea." *Hawaii Journal of Medicine & Public Health* 73, Suppl. 3 (2014): 26–28.

Duponte, Kai, Tammy Martin, Noreen Mokuau, and Lynette Paglinawan. "'Ike Hawai'i—A Training Program for Working with Native Hawaiians." *Journal of Indigenous Voices in Social Work* 1 (2010): 1–24.

Duran, Eduardo. *Healing the Soul Wound: Counseling with American Indians and Other Native Peoples*. New York: Teachers College Press, 2006.

Einhaeuser, Evelyn. "Eduaro Duran: Healing the Soul Wound." *Synergies in Healing Journal* (2015), http://www.synergies-journal.com/synergies/2015/4/2/eduardo-duran-overcoming-historical-trauma. Accessed May 31, 2015.

Fast, Elizabeth, and Delphine Collin-Vezina. "Historical Trauma, Race-based Trauma and Resilience of Indigenous Peoples: A Literature Review." *First Peoples Review* 5 (2010): 126–136.

Felitti, Vincent, Robert Anda, Dale Nordenberg, David Williamson, Alison Spitz, Valerie Edward, Mary Koss, and James Marks. "Relationship of Childhood Abuse and Household Dysfunction to Many of the Leading Causes of Death in Adults. The Adverse Childhood Experiences (ACE) Study." *American Journal of Preventive Medicine* 14 (1998): 245–258.

Hixon, Allen, and Gregory Maskarinec. "Declaration of Alma Ata on Its Thirtieth Anniversary: The Relevance for Family Medicine Today." *Family Medicine* 40 (2008): 584–587.

Hixon, Allen, Seiji Yamada, Paul Farmer, and Gregory Maskarinec. "Social Justice: The Heart of Medical Education." *Social Medicine* 7 (2013): 153–160.

Kamaka, Martina. "Cultural Immersion in a Cultural Competency Curriculum." *Academic Medicine* 76 (2001): 512.

———. "Designing a Cultural Competency Curriculum: Asking the Stakeholders." *Hawaii Medical Journal* 69, Suppl. 3 (2010): 31–34.

———. "Native Hawaiian Health Past, Present, Future: The Genesis of a Course." In *Leaders in Indigenous Medical Education Network 2013, LIME Good Practice Case Studies*, vol. 2. Melbourne: Onemda VicHealth Koori Health Unit, University of Melbourne, 2013, 5–9.

Kamaka, Martina, and N. Emmett Aluli. "Utilizing Cultural Immersion in a Cultural Competency Curriculum: A Conference Report." *Pacific Health Dialog* 8 (2001): 423–428.

Kamaka, Martina, Diane Paloma, and Gregory Maskarinec. "Recommendations for Medical Training: A Native Hawaiian Patient Perspective." *Hawaii Medical Journal* 71, Suppl. 2 (2011): 20–25.

LCME (Liaison Committee on Medical Education). "Functions and Structure of a Medical School: Standards for Accreditation of Medical Education Programs Leading to the M.D. Degree." http://www.lcme.org/publications.htm. Accessed October 8, 2015.

Napier, David, Clyde Ancarno, Beverley Butler, Joseph Calabrese, and Angel Chater, et al. "Culture and Health." *The Lancet* 384 (2014): 1607–1639.

Paglinawan, Richard Likeke. "Ho'oponopono." Lecture at the John A. Burns School of Medicine. September 1, 2009.

Phillips, Gregory. *Addictions and Healing in Aboriginal Country*. Canberrra: Aboriginal Studies Press, 2003, 1–210.

Pukui, Mary Kawena. *'Ōlelo No'eau: Hawaiian Proverbs & Poetical Sayings*. Honolulu: Bishop Museum Press, 1983.

Smedley, Brian. *Unequal Treatment: Confronting Racial and Ethnic Disparities in Health Care*. Washington, DC: Institute of Medicine of the National Academy Press, 2002.

Sotero, Michelle. "A Conceptual Model of Historical Trauma: Implications for Public Health Practice and Research." *Journal of Health Disparities Research and Practice* 1 (2006): 93–108.

Stein, Terry, Ed Krupat, and Richard Frankel. "Talking with Patients. Using the Four Habits Model." The Permanente Medical Group, Physician Education and Development, 2011. http://kpsaccme.com/CME/PPI/PPI_Handout1_Stein_17.pdf. Accessed October 9, 2015.

Tervalon, Melanie, and Jann Murray-García. "Cultural Humility versus Cultural Competence: A Critical Distinction in Defining Physician Training Outcomes in Multicultural Education." *Journal of Health Care for the Poor and Underserved* 9 (1998): 117–125.

U.S. Department of Health and Human Services Office of Minority Health. *Assuring Cultural Competence in Health Care: Recommendations for National Standards and Outcomes-Focused Research Agenda.* Washington, DC: U.S. Government Printing Office, 2000.

From Kalo to Kauka: Becoming a Native Hawaiian Physician

Malia-Susanne Lee, Benjamin Young, Courtney Kielemaikalani Gaddis, Nina Leialoha Beckwith, Sasha Naomi Kehaulani Hayashi Treschuk Fernandes, and Winona Kaalouahi Mesiona Lee

Reflections from the Native Hawaiian Center of Excellence by Malia-Susanne Lee

One of my first duties as the new director of the Native Hawaiian Center of Excellence (NHCOE) was to attend Queen Emma's birthday celebration at The Queen's Medical Center. During the ceremony, I learned how Queen Emma and King Kamehameha IV established the Queen's Hospital. The Native Hawaiian population had been decimated by illness following the arrival of foreign explorers, merchants, and settlers. In 1836, the king and queen went door to door to increase awareness of illness and to garner support for the establishment of a new hospital. In 1859, the Queen's Hospital was built with donations and support of the community, catalyzed by the aloha that our ali'i (royalty) had for all Kānaka Maoli (Native Hawaiians). Today, NHCOE continues to honor our beloved ali'i and meets its mission to improve the physical and mental health of all Native Hawaiians by promoting the success of current and future Native Hawaiian health professionals. NHCOE leads programs in our schools and communities to provide culturally competent educational, research, and service opportunities to Native Hawaiian students and faculty who are committed to improving the health of the people of Hawai'i. Following in the footsteps of NHCOE's former leaders, Drs. Benjamin Young, Nanette Judd, and Winona Mesiona Lee, I embrace my kuleana (responsibility) to inspire and guide the next generation of Native Hawaiian physicians.

NHCOE's primary initiatives include recruiting Native Hawaiian students to enter the field of medicine and other health professions. In 2010, Drs. Nanette Judd and Winona Mesiona Lee created the Native Hawaiian Student Pathways to Medicine Program. Believing that it was instrumental to solidify a pathway for Native Hawaiian students to succeed, they created this program as a hui (group) for Native Hawaiians to engage with students and faculty mentors during their long and sometimes arduous journey to medicine.

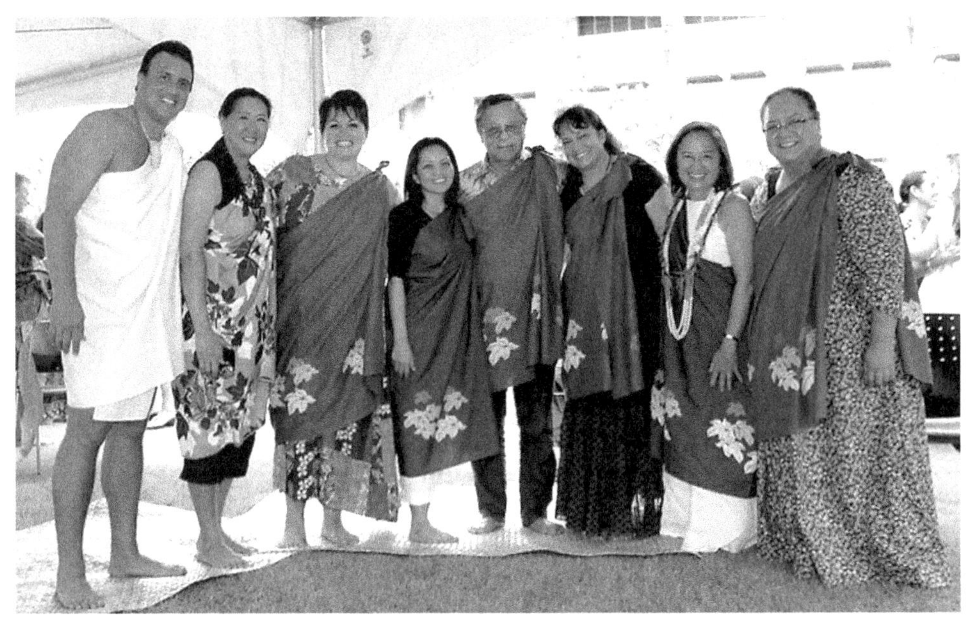

Figure 7.1. 'Awa ceremony for Ahu Ola dedication, 2014. From l to r: Keawe Kaholokula, Marjorie Mau, Dee-Ann Carpenter, Winona Mesiona Lee, Ben Young, Martina Kamaka, Mele Look, and Naleen Andrade. Photo by Chung-Eun Ha, used with permission.

Dr. Sasha Fernandes, NHCOE's health professions recruiter/counselor, leads each hui in a series of workshops to build students' knowledge and confidence to become strong applicants for health profession schools. The program teaches effective learning and study skills, counsels students on academic and professional components related to careers in medicine, and provides financial support for medical college admissions test (MCAT) preparation. More importantly, it honors the cultural strengths of our Native Hawaiian students and imparts wisdom gained from our ancestors that allow students to believe that they are capable of succeeding in their aspiration to become physicians.

Before starting at NHCOE, I had the great pleasure of interviewing Dr. Ben Young. When I asked him about the early days of NHCOE he explained that the route for Native Hawaiians to enter medicine would have been far more difficult had it not been for the 'Imi Ho'ōla program and the Native Hawaiian Center of Excellence. Back in the 1970s many were upset that affirmative action programs were gaining momentum. Many worried that allowing for the admittance of students with lower grade point averages and scores would create a substandard generation of physicians. Concerns about maintaining the standards of the medical school arose. We now know that high admission scores and grade point averages do not always make the best physicians but may be an indication of whether or not someone can pass the courses once they get accepted. It turns out that creating a minimum acceptable grade point average and admission score allowed for an increased diversity of medical school students and enabled some of the first Hawaiians to attend medical school. Studies also show that a diverse physician workforce helps to reduce health inequities related to cultural diversity.

The reflections that follow take us into the lives of Native Hawaiian physicians and physicians-in-training who have been guided by NHCOE. Our hope is that these *mo'olelo* (stories) will inspire our keiki and 'ohana to believe in themselves and to know that a career in the health professions is not only possible but vital if we are to impact the health of Kānaka Maoli. Dr. Ben Young is one of the key leaders in the formation of the Native Hawaiian Center of Excellence and 'Imi Ho'ōla programs and begins the reflections by sharing his own story about how he became a doctor.

Divine Intervention by Benjamin Young

I did not do very well in high school. In fact, I flunked out and had to go to summer school at Roosevelt. I was the youngest of nine children in a family that had no money. High school was difficult mainly because the motivation was not there and college did not appear to be a viable option. My father was a janitor who had a stroke and became completely disabled when I was in the third grade. My mother worked at the cannery as a pineapple trimmer, and my post–high school plans were to work at the Dole Cannery. The one thing that I had in my favor was a willingness to work hard.

Fortunately for me, the minister of the Kaimuki Christian Church was a very significant mentor and advised me that I had potential and wanted to assist me in going to college. This minister, Carl Clark, arranged to get me into a small college in Kentucky even though I lacked the usual acceptable entrance exam scores and possessed an abysmal grade point average. I had no money but arrangements were made for me to work full time at the college, and this work paid for my tuition, room, and board. After two years, I transferred to another small school in Tennessee, Milligan College, where I graduated with a degree in English literature. It was there my wife and I met, and following graduation, DeDe and I were married, and I decided to pursue a career in medicine. The next five years were quite onerous since I never completed any of the pre-med courses. Our first child was born during this period. I began taking classes such as algebra, trigonometry, geometry, biology, chemistry, comparative anatomy, embryology, and physics.

Fortunately, I did well and was offered a scholarship to attend Howard University College of Medicine in Washington, DC. My wife and I loaded up our belongings in a 14-foot U-Haul trailer and began the difficult trek to DC, where after four years of medical school, I received my medical degree. Howard University is one of many historically Black colleges and universities and was founded in 1867 shortly after the Civil War. In the mid-1960s, there were concerns that the nation was facing a severe shortage of physicians, so Congress passed several pieces of legislation to increase health manpower in the country by providing capitation grants for the building of new medical schools, by funding existing medical schools to increase enrollment, and making available more scholarships to encourage students to enter the health professions. I was one of those fortunate to have been a recipient of a scholarship at the time.

During my last year of medical school, I had planned for a residency in either ophthalmology or dermatology. However, that winter, the thermometer dropped to 12 degrees below zero for a two-week period. It was then I realized that it was time to head back home to Hawai'i! I contacted the new chairman of psychiatry, John McDermott, MD, and, after questioning me about my interests, my background, and why I wanted to do a residency in Hawai'i, he asked me about my ethnicity. When I told him I was Hawaiian Chinese, he was startled and said, "Do you know there are no Hawaiians in psychiatry?" Following that conversation with Dr. McDermott, my path was paved, my application for psychiatric residency was approved, and I moved home to Hawai'i.

Shortly after I began my residency, I was contacted by the well-known artist Herb Kawainui Kane about a project to help celebrate Hawai'i's contribution to the founding of this nation. He wanted to build a canoe true to ancient Polynesian design, and sail that canoe to Tahiti and back to Hawai'i without any modern navigational instruments. This was at the earliest beginnings when the Polynesian Voyaging Society was formed and the voyaging canoe *Hōkūle'a* was built. During this period in the early 1970s, there was a tremendous resurgence in love of Hawaiian culture especially in areas such as music, language, and in the 'āina. The book *Nana I Ke Kumu,* the immersion language schools, and Kaho'olawe were focal points of a rising rejuvenation and pride in things Hawaiian. *Hōkūle'a* became an integral part of this Hawaiian renaissance. I was part of the first voyage of *Hōkūle'a* in 1976 as a physician, and since that time so many of JABSOM's graduates have become a vital part of every journey of *Hōkūle'a.* The name of the current voyage, *Mālama Honua,* calls attention to worldwide awareness of the need to take care of our planet, just as our ancestors did, and assure its preservation and continuity for our descendants. Many of our medical school graduates continue to serve with *Hōkūle'a* in their effort to increase worldwide awareness of the need to take care of this planet and its people.

Charting My Own Course by Courtney Kielemaikalani Gaddis

Since I was a little girl, I have always had a deep desire to make a difference in peoples' lives. At about six years of age, I was the goalie on my soccer team. During a game, a girl on the other team tripped and hurt herself. Instead of blocking the goal, I ran out to help her, and her team ended up scoring a goal. It just so happened that we lost that game by one goal. My mom was a little upset that I had left the goal, but she praised me for my caring and nurturing character and recognized how much I didn't like seeing others suffer.

I often thought about what I wanted to be when I grew up. Being a doctor was my ultimate dream, but I didn't know if I was smart enough. Over the years, I developed a deep love for children, and I find myself most happy when I am able to help kids. It is from this love that I was inspired to start my pathway to become a pediatrician.

My ability to help children motivates me. When I was twenty, I signed up for the National Bone Marrow Donor Registry. I worried that my twelve different ethnicities—Japanese, Chinese, Filipino, Portuguese, Hawaiian, Spanish, English, Irish, French, Scotch, American Indian, and Greek—would make me an unlikely match for a patient. Two years later, I matched with a four-year-old boy with leukemia, and I donated my bone marrow to save his life. I had heard that the process of donating would be painful, but I had no hesitations. In fact, despite the pain, it was the most rewarding and eye-opening experience for me. I would do it all again in a heartbeat.

Since the transplant, I have heard that the recipient is doing great and has exceeded doctors' expectations in his recovery and adaptation to the new bone marrow. This little boy is my hero because of all the tribulations he has had to face at such a young age. His fight against adversity inspires me. If I could meet this amazing boy I would tell him that he has given more to me than I could have ever given to him. My experience as a donor has deepened my motivation to help other children who are fighting diseases. As a second-year medical student, I always encourage everyone in my community to sign up with the National Bone Marrow Donor Registry so that more lives can be saved.

I had always known that getting into medical school was going to be difficult. As a student athlete at the University of Hawai'i at Mānoa I spent much of my time on the basketball court. Because of the time commitment with sports, my health-care experience was limited. During the summers I shadowed a pediatrician but continued to worry that other students applying for medical school had more exposure to medicine. I doubted my competitiveness as an applicant. In my junior year of college, I learned about the Native Hawaiian

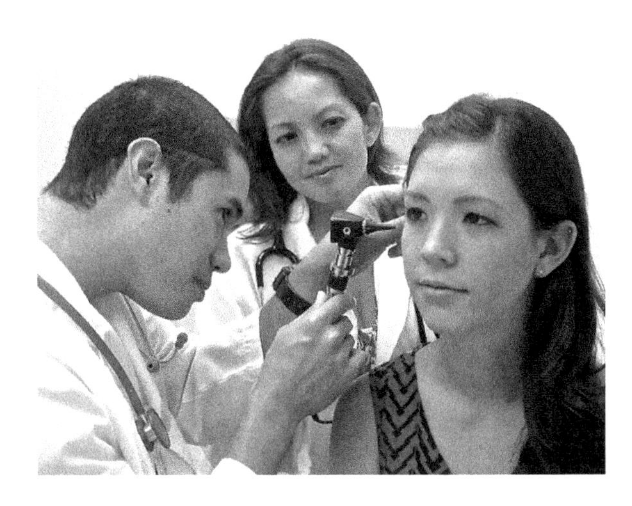

Figure 7.2. Practicing clinical skills, 2012. From left to right: Laua'e Gouveia, Winona Mesiona Lee, and Courtney Gaddis. Photo by Terry Gerber, used with permission.

Student Pathway to Medicine Program through the Native Hawaiian Center of Excellence. I applied and was accepted. There, I gained the skills and experience I needed to build my confidence before applying to medical school. The program supported and guided me on my own pathway and, most important, helped me develop strong relationships with the NHCOE program administrators who have become like family to me. I now share a unique experience with other Native Hawaiian Pathway students who strive to serve the community.

During the Pathways Program, I applied to medical school and I learned about and applied to the 'Imi Hō'ola Post-Baccalaureate Program. I cried when I got my rejection letter from medical school but I prayed that 'Imi Hō'ola would give me a chance. After what seemed like a lifetime of waiting, I was notified of my acceptance into the 'Imi Hō'ola program for the class of 2012–2013. If I could relate the pain of donating bone marrow to the painful process of learning how to be a great medical student in 'Imi Ho'ōla I would say the 'Imi Ho'ōla program was a thousand times more difficult. Through both experiences I learned that I am willing to endure a time of brief pain and suffering for the reward of fulfilling a lifelong dream. I am the first person in my family to go into the medical field, so naturally my family beamed when I completed 'Imi Ho'ōla and matriculated into the JABSOM class of 2017. One thing I take away from my experience with 'Imi Ho'ōla is a strong desire to continue to serve my community. I take pride in my Native Hawaiian heritage and I want to provide health care in underserved communities throughout the Islands. I look forward to being a part of the solution for health inequalities for Native Hawaiians and other Pacific Islanders in my future service as a physician.

Ke Akua, Ka ʻOhana a me Ke Ala Paʻa: God, Family, and the Path
by Nina Leialoha Beckwith

> I'm standing over my cadaver when our teacher yells, "You have one minute. You may begin!" I look down at the man who generously donated his body to our medical school for this very purpose. I nicknamed him Mr. J. I quickly whisper, "Hello Mr. J. Thank you again." The nerves protruding from the vertebrae in his neck are exposed. I look at the question on my anatomy test that reads, "Identify the structure with the pink thread." 45 seconds. With a racing heart I search for the pink thread. It is gently wrapped around a nerve coming from his cervical spine. 30 seconds. Staring at the nerve suddenly forces my attention to a conversation I had with my mom just a few days prior. "I am having surgery on the nerves in my cervical spine," she states in a trembling voice. "I'm really nervous about my throat swelling again." 20 seconds...

I have always had a deep desire to be a healer, a passion largely influenced by my mother. When I was twelve years old, my mom was diagnosed with hepatitis C, and she has gone through many valleys on her journey to restored health. When I was in middle school she had a severe anaphylactic reaction and was rushed by ambulance to the emergency room. She recalls, "When I was in the ER, the doctors lost my heartbeat three times and my throat swelled out to my chin. I was sure I was going to suffocate to death." Ever since, she has suffered from posttraumatic stress disorder (PTSD). A simple cough or mild itchiness in her throat is enough to trigger severe anxiety and shortness of breath. Many patients, like my mom, often don't need sedatives or medications for their condition, but instead they need compassionate, patient, and trustworthy health-care providers to address their deepest needs.

My journey to medicine has taught me how fundamental these qualities are for a future physician and has given me a better idea of the kind of healer I want to be. After graduating from Kalaheo High School in 2005, I was blessed with a ten-year scholarship through the Bill and Melinda Gates Foundation that allowed me to attend the University of California, Davis. Leaving home was rough, but as I left, I reflected on the words of my kumu hula, who always said that every individual has a kuleana (responsibility) to use their unique skills to honor their ancestors and mālama (care for) others. These words were key as I searched for "my place" as a healer. My desire to be a physician continued to grow in college as I served as a peer counselor for a program that supports students from disadvantaged backgrounds. One student I mentored was a young woman who developed PTSD from being sexually assaulted as a child. To help her conquer her fear and frequent hallucinations, a team of professionals treated her holistically, addressing physical symptoms as well as psychosocial ones. Over the next few years, she showed marked improvement in her symptoms. It was deeply rewarding to see how trust and compassion contributed to the beginning of her healing process. Witnessing her care has taught me how determinants of health and access to resources can impact an individual's wellness. My experience as a peer counselor helped me realize that my kuleana was to empower disadvantaged families, especially other Hawaiian families, through health care and education. I decided to move back home to O'ahu to reestablish my roots before entering medical school.

In 2010, I applied for the Teach for America Hawai'i Program and accepted a teaching position at Wai'anae Intermediate School. While teaching full time, I simultaneously attended the University of Hawai'i at Mānoa to earn a master's of education in teaching degree. Teaching was one of the most influential experiences on my journey to medicine. I taught six life science classes, each with an average of thirty seventh grade students. I learned, while teaching in Wai'anae, that barriers to health and success for many students and their families are rooted in disparities in the health-care and education systems. I often saw families feeding their children off the dollar menu at McDonald's because of its affordability. Like the students I counseled in college, many of my students in Wai'anae faced domestic violence and substance abuse in their homes and were in need of support services. I realized there are a plethora of socioeconomic and educational challenges that contribute to poor health trends and outcomes on the Wai'anae Coast. While these challenges were daunting at times, I was inspired on a daily basis by my students' genuine love for their community and their drive to make it a better place.

I started to build connections with the NHCOE at the John A. Burns School of Medicine. I met Dr. Sasha Fernandes, my primary mentor through the Native Hawaiian Student Pathway to Medicine Program. In three years, Dr. Sasha fostered a genuine relationship with me and encouraged me to pursue medical school. She connected me with Native Hawaiian and indigenous physicians, including Dr. Dee-Ann Carpenter, Dr. Lisa Kahikina, Dr. Kelli-Ann Voloch, Dr. Martina Kamaka, Dr. Vanessa Wong, Dr. Winona Mesiona Lee, and more. These individuals and other staff members of the Pathways program became 'ohana to me. The support and encouragement I received from the Native Hawaiian Center of Excellence helped me to believe that I could have a home at the medical school. Inspired by their genuine efforts in the community and their compassion for the patients and the students they mentored, I applied to medical school and was successfully accepted into the University of Hawai'i John A. Burns School of Medicine. I believe that serving as a healer is my calling and my path to building health and hope in our community. I also know that our Akua (God) has a plan for each of us. My desire is to improve the wellness of Native Hawaiians comprehensively, addressing patient needs through culturally sensitive clinical treatment while empowering patients through education. As I continue on this journey, I will always remember the words of my kupuna, who said, "The practice of medicine is the privilege to care." It takes a whole community to build health. I am honored to be a part of the team.

> I quickly shake my head and refocus my attention to my anatomy exam. "10 seconds," our teacher yells. I scribble an answer and rotate stations. After my exam, I call my mom. She has fears and questions about her surgery and writes them all down to ask the surgeon during her next appointment. I hope the surgeon is patient enough to answer all her questions. Three weeks later, here I am, sitting in the surgery waiting room as they operate on her spinal cord. Before she went into the OR the anesthesiologist looked at me holding her hand and with a caring smile said, "Your mom is in good hands. I'll do my best to make sure she is safe and comes out well." In that moment I felt the impact of this trust and the reassuring comfort of compassion. At the end of the day, patients and their families may forget the things you say and the things you do, but they will never forget how you made them feel. My personal mission as a healer is to do everything I can to address the needs of my patients and to do it with a pono (having integrity) heart.

The Accidental Doctor by Malia-Susanne Lee

I was a farm girl growing up so I never thought of becoming a doctor. When I was six, my parents surprised us by moving the family from the suburbs into the country while my siblings and I were visiting our grandparents. My father bought his dream home on a two-acre lot where he could farm home crops and raise his animals and kids. I grew up in my father's own little labor camp where I was the eldest mini–farm hand of three children. My father was a teacher and tended the crops and animals in the afternoons when he returned home, and my mother was a retail manager. My childhood was spent in the school of hard knocks learning the ethics of hard work in the context of planting and harvesting the fields and raising our livestock for slaughter. I'm not sure if I resented having to work hard, but I did resent my father for his strict, no-nonsense, work-and-results-driven ethic.

When I was fourteen my father's kidneys failed and he had to go on hemodialysis. In the midst of his health challenges I was a terrible teen. One day, I got so sassy I just exploded in rage. At the height of my rant I realized that my reaction was so overblown. I felt so selfish and dishonorable that I opened the just-slammed door to my room and apologized to my father, promising to never be disrespectful again. That year, my father had a kidney transplant from his identical twin brother, and I was forever indebted to the team of doctors who gave me a second chance to have a better relationship with my father.

I don't recall thinking about what I wanted to be until the end of high school when my mother forced me to apply for college and scholarships. Even then I got it wrong. The high school guidance counselor told me I was not ready to apply to a university and recommended community college. I was good at math and was told by others that engineers excel in math, so, despite my counselor's advice, I applied to the University of Hawai'i, where I was accepted into the college of electrical engineering. By the end of my first semester and eighteen credits later, I decided engineering was not for me. I did not want to deal with circuitry and binary math. I decided I wanted to work with people.

After withdrawing from engineering I remained undeclared for two years, pondering. Once again, I went to the career counseling center and this time I was told that I should prepare for a career as an administrator or secretary. I learned a great deal about myself while I was sitting in corridors and offices waiting for meetings with my professors and counselors. I was unknowingly developing my listening and problem-solving skills that are so essential to medicine. In those hallways and waiting room chairs total strangers would plop themselves next to me and start telling me their stories of worry and pain. I would listen quietly, just thinking of words I could offer that would possibly make a difference in their situations and they would leave with a smile on their face. Looking back, it should not surprise me that I had fallen into this medical career where strangers walk through the door with problems that I work to find solutions for.

Once I received my biology degree, I had no idea what to do with it. I was not interested in lab work, I felt that I wasn't smart enough to be a doctor, and I had not prepared myself to be a teacher. I went home to my parents and back to work at our local grocery store. The following semester, my younger sister graduated after just three years at her university and was heading to law school on the fast track, leaving me in the dust. Not wanting to be outdone, I decided that I would seriously look into the option of medical school.

I grew up with only a few health-care role models and had no idea what it would take to become a doctor. The only doctors I had ever known were my pediatrician and my next-door neighbor's father, who were both very tall white males. I'd seen a female doctor once on a television show, but the idea of a female physician was absurd to me. Though my grandmother was a nurse, I had no understanding of what being a health-care provider meant. In college I heard of other women pursuing medicine and thought the idea was absurd.

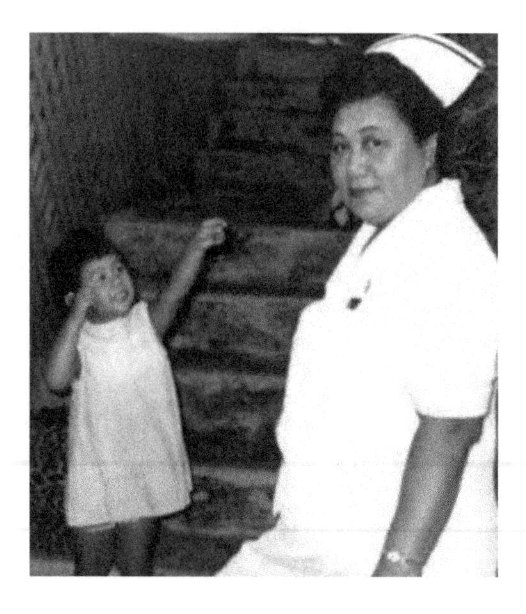

Figure 7.3. Malia-Susanne Lee with her grandmother Susanne Lui Kwan Medeiros, one of the first Native Hawaiian nurses from the University of Hawai'i, 1971. Photo by Daphne Lee, used with permission.

My grandmother Susanne Kapihenui Medeiros would always tell us that she was one of the first Native Hawaiians to graduate from the University of Hawai'i School of Nursing. While she drove us around town, she would point out the neighborhoods in Kalihi and Pālolo where she would go door to door giving children their immunizations, and we would often visit her at Lē'ahi Hospital, where she worked. I recall once asking my grandmother if she felt bad for having to give shots to the children and making them cry. She looked at me surprised and said, "Of course not, those shots are saving their lives." I realize now that she was doing her best to reduce the incidence of illness and health disparities that once plagued the native peoples of Hawai'i.

As I researched medical school admission requirements, I stumbled upon the 'Imi Ho'ōla Post-Baccalaureate Program at the University of Hawai'i John A. Burns School of Medicine. The 'Imi Ho'ōla program is designed to help underrepresented students develop the skills they needed to get into medical school. I applied and was accepted. In 'Imi Ho'ōla, I was immersed in a world of academic challenge and competition that I had never experienced before. It was the most difficult time of my entire academic life, but I learned to focus and to pay attention to details. Thankfully, I did well in the program and was later accepted into medical school at the University of Hawai'i John A. Burns School of Medicine.

My time spent with 'Imi Ho'ōla helped me to forge a commitment to the people of Hawai'i through service in primary care. The beginning of my career was spent turning a teen health and OB/GYN clinic into a family practice clinic for the community health center. Many of my first patients were teenage and adult females who came in day after day to discuss family planning, pregnancy prevention, and solutions to their challenging situations. To break the monotony of seeing people for the same type of problems, I found it helpful to understand my patients' lives in the context of their visits. I was most troubled by teenagers who came in focused on friends and foolishness at the expense of their education and high school completion. I began to wonder if there was anything I could say that would make a difference in their lives, and how I could make an impact on a larger number of adolescents as opposed to one patient at a time. As I continued working at the clinic, the teenagers became adults who developed predictable and anticipated life struggles.

My practice went on as usual. Often, I'd think about the thousands of strangers who had walked into my office during my years of practice. It was my job to figure out why they were there and what I could do for them in fifteen minutes or less. Managing the social aspects affecting patient wellness was one of my greatest challenges. It was difficult for me to understand why most people couldn't find answers to their own problems. No matter how many times I would offer a solution, the same problems would often remain.

I began to wonder if my expertise might be more useful in a global or community setting. I understand now that although medicine may have a scientific basis of diagnostic algorithms and evidence-based delivery-of-care models, the fact remains that a less predictable human element must be considered in every case in order to help people heal. That less predictable element can include a person's relationships, environment, struggles, or spiritual well-being.

I decided to transition my career toward academics, and I pursued the fellowship in medical research and education through the Native Hawaiian Center of Excellence. My focus was to give back to the Native Hawaiian community by improving the health awareness of adolescents with an emphasis on education and cultural awareness. After learning more about traditional Hawaiian healing and *ho'oponopono* (the practice of reconciliation and forgiveness) by kūpuna such as the Paglinawans, I am reaffirmed in my belief that from the Native Hawaiian perspective, healing is 10 percent medicinal and 90 percent spiritual. Bringing all things that impact one's life to the table is essential to healing. In medical school, I recall very distinctly being told that understanding a patient's religion is an important factor in patient care, but that my own religion had no role. Confused, I mistakenly equated religion with spirituality, which inevitably emerges in the course of daily patient interactions. Understanding traditional Hawaiian healing has helped me to bridge the disconnect that sometimes exists between spiritual and physical healing. Spirituality transcends religion and can sometimes be the broken bulb that when fixed will shed light on patients' illness and well-being. Understanding this connection lets me know that I am exactly where I am supposed to be.

My role as NHCOE director has allowed me to work with some of Hawai'i's fantastic leaders and innovators in education, Native Hawaiian culture, and health. During an NHCOE planning session with the founder of Nā Pua No'eau, Dr. David Sing (affectionately known as Uncle David), he said, "We are not reaching for children who know they want to be doctors. We are reaching for those who don't know and are helping them see who they *could* be." I was one of those children. I had no intention of becoming a doctor when I was in high school and was unaware of the Uncle Davids in my life—though as I look back they were certainly there.

Conclusion

These pathway reflections demonstrate the compassion, altruism, and perseverance of our current and future Native Hawaiian physicians. We celebrate the accomplishments of all our students and highlight the importance of mentors, family, and friends while on their journey. For nearly twenty-five years, NHCOE has guided Native Hawaiian students through the challenges of becoming physicians and has proven to be an instrumental source of support for students on their path to becoming healers for their communities. NHCOE is committed to supporting aspiring *kauka* (doctors) reach their career goals through programs like the Native Hawaiian Student Pathway to Medicine Program. Over the past five years, eighty-four students have enrolled in the Native Hawaiian Student Pathway to Medicine, and many of them have been successful in their pursuit of careers in medicine. As our students become doctors, teaching faculty, and future health-care leaders, they also become the future mentors for generations to come. We encourage all kauka to continue to share their mo'olelo that inspire the coming generations to explore health careers and to encourage them to become a part of the legacy that is the Native Hawaiian Center of Excellence.

The authors would like to thank the Hawai'i State Legislature and the U.S. Department of Health and Human Services, Bureau of Health Workforce, Health Resources and Services Administration (HRSA) for their support of the Native Hawaiian Center of Excellence.

This program is supported by the Bureau of Health Workforce, Health Resources and Services Administration (HRSA) of the U.S. Department of Health and Human Services (HHS) under the University of Hawai'i Center of Excellence Grant number D34HP16044. The information, content and conclusions are those of the authors and should not be construed as the official position or policy of, nor should any endorsements be inferred by, HRSA, HHS, or the U.S. government.

Community and Research Together

Claire Townsend Ing, Rebecca Delafield, and Shelley Soong

Native Hawaiians have faced historical and cultural traumas leading to modern-day inequities in the social, economic, and political realms. These inequities contribute to poor health status for many Native Hawaiians. Two groups have attempted to improve these health outcomes, academic researchers and the Native Hawaiian community. However, oftentimes the approaches and goals of these two groups may not complement each other. Community-Based Participatory Research (CBPR) is an approach that seeks to combine community goals, action, and priorities with those of academic research. This chapter illustrates the evolution of CBPR in Hawai'i, and its meaningful principles that have been effective for both Native Hawaiian and research communities.

Health Status of Native Hawaiians

Historic and contemporary changes to the social fabric, contact with other cultures, and the resulting cultural trauma have had severe economic, environmental, and educational impacts on the Native Hawaiian community.[1,2] These social factors work to, in part, determine the physical health of Native Hawaiians as described by Dr. Kaholokula earlier in this monograph. The poor economic, environmental, and educational indicators experienced by many Native Hawaiians have all been associated with poor health outcomes and are reflected in the current health status of the Native Hawaiian community.

Almost 38 percent of Native Hawaiians are living at or below the poverty line.[3,4] Native Hawaiians are more likely to live in neighborhoods that do not promote healthy lifestyles,[5] and nearly half of Native Hawaiian households experience problems of affordability, overcrowding, or structural inadequacy.[6] Native Hawaiians also struggle with educational attainment, another indicator of socioeconomic status. Compared to other major ethnic groups in Hawai'i, Native Hawaiian students continue to score lower in both standardized reading and math assessments.[7] Additionally, when compared to the general population of Hawai'i, Native Hawaiians are not only less likely to have a bachelor's degree, with only 15 percent of Native Hawaiians and other Pacific Islanders holding at least a bachelor's degree,[8] but are also less likely to be employed in high-paying management and professional occupations.[9]

These economic, environmental, and educational struggles are reflected in the poor health status of Native Hawaiians. Compared to other ethnic groups in Hawai'i, Native Hawaiians have higher rates of death and are dying at younger ages,[10,11] they have a greater risk for developing and dying from cancer,[12,13] and they have a higher prevalence of obesity, diabetes, asthma, hypertension, and heart disease.[14] In addition, Native Hawaiians have the second highest rate of diagnosed HIV infection and the second shortest AIDS survival rate of all Americans.[15]

Community Approach versus Research Approach

Both the research community and the Native Hawaiian community have worked to address these social factors and health outcomes. However, while their approaches may not have been as opposing sides, they certainly have not been in concert. This predicament is illustrated even at a fundamental level, such as the Native Hawaiian and the research communities' differing definitions of health. Traditionally, Native Hawaiians trace their genealogy to the union of Wākea and Papa hānaumoku, the sky father and the earth mother.[16] Each individual is an ancestor of the land and the nature that it contains.[17] When considering this holistic identity, it is not surprising that the Native Hawaiian concept of health and well-being is distinctly connected to the broader physical and spiritual environment. This stands in stark contrast to the definition of health and well-being that has been proffered by the Western medical and academic institutions. The National Institutes of Health, the nation's top medical research agency, has a mission to "seek fundamental knowledge about the nature and behavior of living systems and the application of that knowledge to enhance health, lengthen life, and reduce illness and disability."[18] The concept of health used here is much more centered on biology, an absence of disease, and lengthening of life. This divergence in fundamental perceptions of health creates marked differences in the approaches taken by the Native Hawaiian community and academic researchers to improving health.

Community Approach

Today, a multitude of community-based nonprofit organizations and state programs work to address health, as well as economic, environmental, and cultural revitalization, with a shared mission of improving the well-being of Native Hawaiian communities. Community-initiated actions have established a foundation for addressing health issues and their broader social determinants.

The Native Hawaiian community has responded to assaults and challenges to their land, culture, and physical health in various ways, most notably through community organizing efforts to effect change. Results of these efforts are seen in the creation of new legislation and changes to policies that create new programs, reestablish rights, and protect existing resources. Examples familiar to many include the Protect Kaho'olawe 'Ohana movement,[19] the protests to stop the bombing of Mākua Valley,[20] the struggle of the Waiāhole-Waikāne community to stop development and win land leases from the state, and the reforms from the Constitutional Convention. These reforms established protections for Native Hawaiians to practice their cultural traditions, made the Hawaiian language an official language of Hawai'i (along with English), and established the Office of Hawaiian Affairs.[21] An example of collective action focused on physical health is the work by the E Ola Mau group and the passage of the Native Hawaiian Health Improvement Act in 1988.[22] This act led to the establishment of the Native Hawaiian Health Care System, which includes five organizations on five different islands across the state with a mission to improve the health of Native Hawaiians in their communities.[23,24] These actions by Native Hawaiians to protect and promote health, cultural knowledge and practice, and natural resources were vital steps toward changing the political and social realities of Native Hawaiians. Achievements such as these empower communities, which can result in improvements to overall quality of life.[25]

While these community-driven successes must be recognized for the gains they generated, disparities persist. This does not diminish the work that is done in and by the community, but reflects the scale of the challenges that communities are attempting to address. Additionally, community programs or coalitions may fluctuate in terms of their ability or interest in addressing issues, especially if the "problem" fades from the spotlight.[26] Other obstacles facing community-based organizations include funding shortages, decentralized communities, limited capacity to fully implement and sustain efforts, and lack of data to monitor improvements.[27,28]

Health Research Approach

Public health and medical research are also trying to address these inequities. Health and medical research have contributed immensely to improved health globally and locally (e.g., vaccines, sanitation, and penicillin). Research relies on observation, measurement, and experimentation to uncover new knowledge. Observation and measurement produce data that can help us understand population health trends, disease progression, behavioral risk factors, etc. Data for Native Hawaiians can reveal health concerns and draw attention to issues, which can result in increased research and programmatic funds to address the identified health concerns. In 1997, the Office of Management and Budget changed their standard regulations for the collection of race and ethnic data so that the category of Asian American and Pacific Islanders was disaggregated into Native Hawaiian and Other Pacific Islander versus Asian American.[29] Research examining disaggregated data uncovered differences in cancer rates between Asian Americans and Native Hawaiian and other Pacific Islanders.[30] Studies also showed differences in incidents and trends in certain cancers between Native Hawaiian and other Pacific Islander subgroups.[31] Understanding the variations in disease rates aids in the development of more effective prevention and treatment strategies for different populations.[32]

Health research can also help design interventions that treat or prevent disease, and determine their effectiveness. The Diabetes Prevention Project was a watershed clinical research trial that supplied evidence showing that a lifestyle intervention (which focused on changes to diet and increased physical activity) can help prevent or delay the onset of type 2 diabetes in people at high risk for the disease.[33] The study found both a lifestyle intervention and medication (metformin) were effective at delaying the onset of diabetes.[34] However, the lifestyle intervention was superior to the medication in delaying the onset of diabetes.[35] The lifestyle intervention has been successfully adapted for many different community types and populations, including Native Hawaiians, and found to impact weight loss.[36]

There are a number of other examples of the benefit and usefulness of research to address health concerns including improving access, care, and decreasing costs.[37] Yet, while there have been great gains made through scientific advances, there remain disparities in health status between Native Hawaiians and other ethnic/racial groups. One problem is that, on average, it can take seventeen years between the revelation of new knowledge through scientific inquiry and the application of the new knowledge in practice.[38] These difficulties have led health researchers to focus more attention and resources on health disparities research, including looking to community-engaged approaches to research that could create a bridge between health research and impacting health in the community.

Community and Research Joint Approach

Both community groups and academic research are working, albeit from different starting points, with different tools, and using different tactics, toward the same goal. These differences have historically been barriers to integrating community efforts and research. For example, there exist painful examples in the not-so-distant past of egregious transgressions and troublingly unethical treatment of people involved in research.[39] While many advances have been made to protect human subjects in research,[40,41,42] mistrust can be a particular challenge for research projects in indigenous and marginalized communities who have been exploited and harmed in the course of research studies.[43,44]

Another discrepancy between traditional academic research and community is the difference between a controlled setting and a real-world setting, which can influence the usefulness of the intervention.[45] For example an evidence-based intervention that showed promise in a research study may not be practical for implementation in a community clinic setting where conditions are very different—resources or equipment may be limited, and the population may be diverse with a variety of sociocultural, environmental, and socioeconomic factors that impact lives differently than the original research subjects.[46,47,48]

In spite of these challenges, increasingly communities and researchers have been working together and capitalizing on their differences through an approach to research called community-based participatory research (CBPR). CBPR is "a collaborative process that equitably involves all partners in the research process and recognizes the unique strengths that each brings. CBPR begins with a research topic of importance to the community with the aim of combining knowledge and action for social change to improve community health and eliminate health disparities."[49] It is a collaborative, co-equal, partnership approach between the researcher and the community to work to discover solutions to health disparities or challenges within the community.[50,51] While each CBPR partnership varies, there are nine principles to which they strive to adhere.[52] Below, each of these principles is discussed in turn and illustrated by CBPR projects in Hawai'i.

Unit of Identity

Community-based participatory research recognizes the community as a unit of identity. "Community is characterized by a sense of identification and emotional connection to other members, common symbol systems, shared values and norms, mutual—although not necessarily equal—influence, common interests, and commitment to meeting shared needs."[53] In this way, the community in each CBPR project is self-defined. Shiramizu, Milne, Terada, and colleagues worked to increase anal cancer screening in HIV-infected Native Hawaiians, Pacific Islanders, Asians, and disadvantaged and rural populations. Despite the sociodemographic diversity in this study, individual participants' common HIV-positive status creates a sense of identification, emotional connection, and therefore community. Also included in this project were organizations that work with this community (e.g., AIDS service organizations, health-care practitioners, the Hawai'i State Department of Health).[54] Other

CBPR projects work with communities that identify in a variety of ways. The Partnerships for Improving Lifestyle Interventions (PILI) 'Ohana Project is a decade-long CBPR partnership between the Department of Native Hawaiian Health at the John A. Burns School of Medicine, Hawai'i Maoli, Ke Ola Mamo, Kōkua Kalihi Valley, and Kula no na Po'e Hawai'i. The aim of the PILI 'Ohana Project is to address obesity and obesity-related health disparities in Native Hawaiians and other Pacific Islanders. This project conceives of Native Hawaiians and other Pacific Islanders as a community.[55] Additionally, the project has representation from four distinct community-based organizations that serve more specific communities (e.g., Kalihi Valley, a specific homestead, an organization's members). By recognizing the community as a unit of identity and allowing the community to self-identify, CBPR understands and respects the commonalities and differences that are present in our communities.

Build on Strengthens and Resources

The second principle of CBPR is that it seeks to build on strengths and resources within the community. These strengths and resources may include those of individuals, both properties and talents; social networks; and community-based organizations. Recognizing and building on the strengths of the community shifts the paradigm from a deficiency model of communities to a resiliency model. Working together with the community to identify and build on these strengths and resources supports community members' ability to collectively act to improve their health.[56] 'Imi Hale, the Native Hawaiian Cancer Network, has endeavored to identify the strengths and resources in the cancer community, from patients and family members to the Native Hawaiian Health Care System (NHHCS) and Department of Health.[57] They offer training to improve the capacity of the NHHCS to provide cancer-related services, strengthen cancer prevention services of other health care providers, and provide a "research home" for researchers who need housing for their studies. By identifying the strengths and resources present in the cancer-care community, 'Imi Hale works with the community to better enable them to achieve their cancer-care goals. The CBPR project encourages communities and community-based organizations to collaborate. This collaboration can heighten the effectiveness and reach of each community's or community-based organization's efforts.[58]

Collaborative, Equitable Partnerships

Community-based participatory research facilitates collaborative, equitable partnerships in all research phases and involves an empowering and power-sharing process that attends to social inequalities.[59] The community and researchers participate as equal members sharing control throughout the research process, for example, creating the research question, designing the study, collecting data, interpreting the results, and disseminating the results.[60] This shared responsibility creates research projects that are both scientifically sound and relevant to the community. The HELA study,[61] which developed a culturally tailored cardiac rehabilitation program for patients with coronary artery disease, worked to develop a research team that was comprised of individuals with scientific (i.e., health care, health intervention development, and research methodology) and cultural (i.e., cultural protocol and hula) expertise. All team members had influence in the research process, which resulted in discussion and compromises. A commitment to this principle of creating equity across the partnership allowed for conflicts to be resolved and for the collaboration to prosper. This team, with input also from the patient community, was able to create a cardiac rehabilitation program that is grounded in the hula tradition, culturally relevant to participants, and clinically effective.

Balance Research and Action

Community-based participatory research strives to achieve a balance between research and action for the mutual benefits of all partners.[62] These projects should do more than produce knowledge through research; they should also lead to improvements in community health and well-being.[63] The project by Shiramizu, Milne, Terada, and colleagues contributed to our knowledge of anal cancer screening barriers and facilitating factors as well as increasing screening rates in HIV-positive men and women.[64] The PILI 'Ohana Project has contributed to science by advancing our knowledge on weight loss and weight loss maintenance in Native Hawaiian and other Pacific Islander communities.[65] The project has also developed several culturally tailored, evidence-based interventions that are being adopted by community health centers, diabetes educators, and NHHCS across the state. Finally, the project has fostered social change within communities (e.g., increased awareness of health), development of community-based organizations (e.g., improved skills of employees), and personal change for some of the community partners (e.g., furthering education).[66] Community-academic partnerships are an effective approach for the generation of scientific knowledge and improving community health.

Co-learning and Capacity Building

The fifth principle of CBPR is to promote co-learning and capacity building among all partners. Community-based participatory research should actively work to transfer knowledge and skills between partners.[67] The PILI 'Ohana Project illustrates this well. Researchers have learned that differing intervention foci and strategies may be needed for different subpopulations in Native Hawaiian and other Pacific Islanders' communities; lots of interaction, games, activities, and immediate positive reinforcement seem to enhance the weight loss interventions; and community peer educators are able to deliver evidence-based interventions and achieve significant weight loss or improvement in glycemic control for their participants.[68] Additionally, researchers have become more aware of the challenges faced by and priorities of community-based organizations. The community, in turn, has built its knowledge and skill base, becoming more knowledgeable about the research process, and more skilled at grant writing, and having improved negotiation skills in working with other researchers. The partnership offered a variety of capacity-building workshops for this purpose (e.g., database management, research design, behavioral change strategies). When done well, CBPR projects can do more that improve the health of a community or advance scientific knowledge. By promoting co-learning and capacity building, the knowledge and skill base of all partners can improve for the long-term benefit of both.

Cyclical and Iterative Process

The next principle of CBPR is that it is a cyclical and iterative process, which includes partnership development and maintenance, the research process, and any actions or policies aimed at the maintenance of any improvements in well-being gained through the research project.[69] Establishing and maintaining an effective partnership takes considerable time and flexibility. 'Imi Hale's research-review process required that the community be sought and feedback be incorporated into the proposal development process. This process took four months. However, it was through this process that 'Imi Hale researchers were able to strengthen their relationships with community partners.[70] Shiramizu and colleagues engaged with community advisory groups and organizations serving the HIV-positive populations.[71] This interactive feedback was used throughout the research process to improve upon the research design and methods.[72] As an iterative process, CBPR allows both community and academic partners to respond to changing priorities and newly identified challenges or opportunities creating a stronger and more effective partnership.

Addresses Health from a Positive Perspective

The seventh principle of CBPR is that it addresses health from a positive perspective and recognizes and attends to multiple (including social) determinants of health.[73] Addressing health from a positive perspective means that the community and researchers alike emphasize well-being rather than ill health. For instance, the PILI 'Ohana Program encourages healthy lifestyle changes and addresses healthy eating, physical activity, and time and stress management. Participants focus on making positive lifestyle changes rather than focusing on the negative health effects of obesity and related diseases. The recognition that health is influenced by social, community, and political factors leads CBPR projects to strive for social change that will attenuate health disparities. As discussed previously, data on the health of Native Hawaiians and other Pacific Islanders have been obscured for years by the aggregation of their data with that of Asian Americans. The data generated by CBPR, both qualitative and quantitative in nature, has helped to bring these health disparities to light and advocate for a disaggregation of the data across the United States.[74] Additionally, data from these projects also help us to better understand some of the social determinants of health (e.g., lack of culturally appropriate cancer education materials, lack of access to quality physical activity and healthy eating resources).[75,76]

Broad-Based Dissemination of Results

Community-based participatory research does not limit the dissemination of results to traditional academic venues (e.g., conferences and scientific journals); rather it strives to disseminate findings and knowledge gained to all partners and involves all partners in the dissemination process.[77] The dissemination of results includes the use of language that is accessible to and respectful of audiences. The PILI 'Ohana Project has performed a variety of dissemination activities, including the presentation of study results to community leaders, study participants, and the scientific community. Additionally, community members have been involved in the preparation of every manuscript submitted on the PILI 'Ohana Project and have assisted in data interpretation.[78,79,80,81,82,83,84] In this way, CBPR promotes the use of findings throughout the communities involved and discourages "helicopter" research, in which researchers fly into a community, conduct their research, and leave, taking all the results with them.

Long-Term, Iterative Process

The final principle of CBPR is a recognition that it is a long-term process and requires a commitment to sustainability.[85] "Long-term" refers to the development of relationships and commitment that extend beyond the single research project or funding period. The commitment is to the partnership rather that to a specific project. For instance, a CBPR partnership to understand and support the process of disclosure of intimate partner violence continued to meet and communicate after their initial funding period had ended. Their work during this time focused on the generation of additional manuscripts and preparation of new funding proposals including pilot funding that may only be able to support a portion of the partnership.[86] As a long-term process, a successful community-academic partnership requires a commitment by all partners to a common mission and vision for success.[87]

Conclusion

Adherence to these nine principles, and to the collaborative spirit behind the CBPR approach, can result in significant benefits for the academic and community researchers involved as well as to our scientific knowledge base and overall community health and wellness. By engaging the community, the research is more valid and immediately relevant to those whom it is aimed at helping.[88] Participation in CBPR can also strengthen the skills of academic researchers and improve the capacity of the community to effectively address their health and wellness needs.[89] Community-based participatory research also can help to address the needs of marginalized communities by directly examining their needs as they identify them.[90] Other benefits of CBPR include creating theory that is informed by the community, which can in turn lead to more effective practice,[91] help overcome the history of distrust on the part of the community toward research,[92] and help provide funding for community-based programs and employees.[93]

In the face of these benefits, there are also limitations to CBPR. For instance, CBPR recognizes the community as a unit of identity. This can obscure the differences that exist between community members. These differences between communities and community members can lead to disparities in the results for interventions,[94] as well as disagreements and differences in priorities that can threaten the overall partnership.[95] Additional challenges facing researchers interested in CBPR are the structure of many funding organizations and the tenure process at academic institutions. Grant mechanisms that allow for the time it takes to fully engage the community in problem identification, research question development, and proposal planning are extremely rare. Rather, partnerships with the community must be built outside of these funding sources. This limits the money, and therefore time, that is available to both community and academics interested in developing a partnership. In order to progress in their career, academic researchers must engage in "scholarly activity." In many institutions, working with the community is not seen as a scholarly activity and is thus not rewarded in the same way.[96,97]

However, CBPR is iterative and thus involves incremental development. This extends past the partnerships created and into the funding mechanisms and academic institutions. Over time, with continued work, these limitations can be addressed. Community-based participatory research is an approach to research that seeks to place the community and academics on equal footing in the development of knowledge to improve community health and well-being. This approach to research is particularly appropriate for use with communities that have historically been exploited by the research community specifically, but also by society more generally. As a community that has been taken advantage of by researchers in the past, the use of CBPR with Native Hawaiian communities is particularly appropriate. The principles of CBPR elevate the standards of research. By striving to adhere to these nine principles, both community and academic partners can enhance their strengths and limit their weaknesses. The community can increase their overall capacity to provide services to their community members while academic researchers can improve the applicability of the knowledge generated and the reach of their research outputs.

The authors thank the PILI ʻOhana Project participants, community researchers, and staff of the participating community organizations: Hawaiʻi Maoli, The Association of Hawaiian Civic Clubs, Ke Ola Mamo, Kula no na Poʻe Hawaiʻi, and Kōkua Kalihi Valley. This study was supported by the National Institute on Minority Health and Health Disparities (NIMHD) with awards to the PILI ʻOhana Program: Partnerships to Overcome Obesity Disparities in Hawaii (R24MD001660). The authors' time was also supported by NIMHD institutional infrastructure (U54MD007584) and The Queen's Health Systems. The content is solely the responsibility of the authors and does not necessarily represent the official views of the NIMHD, the National Institutes of Health, or The Queen's Health Systems.

NOTES

1. Marc Pilisuk, JoAnn McAllister, and Jack Rothman, "Social Change Professionals and Grassroots Organizing: Functions and Dilemmas," in *Community Organizing and Community Building for Health*, ed. Meredith Minkler (New Brunswick, NJ: Rutgers University Press, 1997).
2. Howard K. Koh, Sarah C. Oppenheimer, Sarah B. Massin-Short, Karen M. Emmons, Alan C. Geller, and Kasisomayajula Viswanath, "Translating Research Evidence into Practice to Reduce Health Disparities: A Social Determinants Approach," *American Journal of Public Health* 100, Suppl. 1 (2010).
3. Adam Wagstaff, "Poverty and Health Sector Inequalities," *Bulletin of the World Health Organization* 80, no. 2 (2002).
4. White House Initiative on Asian Americans and Pacific Islanders, "What You

Should Know about Native Hawaiians and Pacific Islanders," ed. U.S. Department of Education (Washington, DC, 2010).

5. Marjorie K. Mau, Kara N. Wong, Jimmy Efird, Margaret West, Erin P. Saito, and Jay Maddock, "Environmental Factors of Obesity in Communities with Native Hawaiians," *Hawaii Medical Journal* 67, no. 9 (2008).

6. U.S. Department of Housing and Urban Development, "Housing Problems and Needs of Native Hawaiians" (Washington, DC, 1993).

7. Shawn K. Kana'iaupuni, Nolan Malone, and Koren Ishibashi, "Ka Huaka'i: 2005 Native Hawaiian Educational Assessment" (Honolulu: Kamehameha Schools, Pauahi Publications, 2005).

8. US Census Bureau, "Census Bureau Facts for Features: Asian/Pacific American Heritage Month," https://www.census.gov/newsroom/releases/archives/facts_for_features_ special_editions/cb10-ff07.html.

9. Seiji Naya, "Income Distribution and Poverty Alleviation for the Native Hawaiian Community," in *2nd Annual Hawaiian Business Conference* (Honolulu: Office of Hawaiian Affairs, 2007).

10. Sela V. Panapasa, Marjorie K. Mau, David R. Williams, and James W. McNally, "Mortality Patterns of Native Hawaiians across Their Lifespan: 1990–2000," *American Journal of Public Health* 100, no. 11 (2010).

11. Joseph Balabis, Ann Pobutsky, Kathleen K. Baker, Caryn Tottori, and Florentina Salvail, "The Burden of Cardiovascular Disease in Hawaii 2007" (Honolulu: Hawaii State Department of Health, 2007).

12. Lihua Liu, Anne-Michelle Noone, Scarlett Lin Gomez, Steve Scoppa, James T. Gibson, Daphne Lichtensztajn, Kari Fish, Lynne R. Wilkens, Marc T. Goodman, Cyllene Morris, Sandy Kwong, Dennis Deapen, and Barry A. Miller, "Cancer Incidence Trends among Native Hawaiians and Other Pacific Islanders in the United States, 1990–2008," *Journal of the National Cancer Institute* 105, no. 15 (2013).

13. "Health and Health Care of Native Hawaiian and other Pacific Islander Older Adults," retrieved from http://geriatrics.stanford.edu/ethnomed/hawaiian_pacific_islander/. In V. S. Periyakoil, ed. eCampus Geriatrics, Stanford, CA, 2010.

14. Mele A. Look, Mililani K. Trask-Batti, Robert Agres, Marjorie L. Mau, and Joseph K. Kaholokula, "Assessment and Priorities for Health & Well-Being in Native Hawaiians & Other Pacific Peoples" (Honolulu: Center for Native and Pacific Health Disparaties Research, 2013).

15. Stephen Stafford, "Caught between 'the Rock' and a Hard Place: The Native Hawaiian and Pacific Islander Struggle for Identity in Public Health," *American Journal of Public Health* 100, no. 5 (2010).

16. Richard Kekuni Blaisdell, "Historical and Cultural Aspects of Native Hawaiian Health: The Health of Native Hawaiians, a Selective Report on Health Status and Health Care in the 1980's," in *Social Process in Hawaii* (Honolulu: University of Hawai'i Press, 1989).

17. Ibid.

18. National Institutes of Health, "About NIH," http://www.nih.gov/about/mission.htm.

19. Protect Kaho'olawe 'Ohana, "History," http://www.protectkahoolaweohana.org/index.html.

20. Earthjustice, "Down to Earth: David Henkin on Oahu's Makua Valley," http://earthjustice.org/features/down-to-earth-david-henkin-on-oahu-s-makua-valley.

21. Office of Hawaiian Affairs, "History: The Establishment of OHA," http://www.oha.org/about/history/.
22. US Congress, "Native Hawaiian Health Care Act of 1988," in *PL 100-579* (Washington, DC, 1988).
23. Protect Kaho'olawe 'Ohana, "History."
24. Richard Kekuni Blaisdell, "Update on Kanaka Maoli (Indigenous Hawaiian) Health," *Asian American and Pacific Islander Journal of Health* 4, no. 1–3 (1996).
25. Meredith Minker, "Community Organizing Among the Elderly Poor in San Francisco's Tenderloin District," in *Community Organizing and Community Building for Health*, ed. Meredith Minkler (New Brunswick, NJ: Rutgers University Press, 2002).
26. Stephen B. Fawcett, "Some Lessons on Community Organization and Change," in *Reflections on Community Organization: Enduring Themes and Critical Issues*, ed. J. Rothman (Itasca, IL: F. E. Peacock Publishers, 1999).
27. Maile Taualii, Joey Quenga, Raynald Samoa, Salim Samanani, and Doug Dover, "Liberating Data: Accessing Native Hawaiian and Other Pacific Islander Data from National Data Sets," *AAPI Nexus: Policy, Practice, and Community* 9, no. 1 (2011).
28. Abraham Wandersman and Paul Florin, "Community Interventions and Effective Prevention," *American Psychologist* 58, no. 6-7 (2003).
29. Sela Panapasa, Kamana'opono Crabbe, and Joseph Keawe'aimoku Kaholokula, "Efficacy of Federal Data: Revised Office of Management and Budget Standard for Native Hawaiian and Other Pacific Islanders Examined," *AAPI Nexus: Policy, Practice, and Community* 9, no. 1–2 (2011).
30. Anh Bao Nguyen, Neetu Chawla, Anne-Michelle Noone, and Shobha Srinivasan, "Disaggregated Data and Beyond: Future Queries in Cancer Control Research," *Cancer Epidemiology Biomarkers and Prevention* 23, no. 11 (2014).
31. Lihua Liu et al., "Cancer Incidence Trends among Native Hawaiians and Other Pacific Islanders in the United States, 1990–2008."
32. Tessie Guillermo and Shobha Srinivasan, "Toward Improved Health: Disaggregating Asian American and Native Hawaiian/Pacific Islander Data," *American Journal of Public Health* 90, no. 11 (2000).
33. Group Diabetes Prevention Program Research, "Reduction in the Incidence of Type 2 Diabetes with Lifestyle Interventions or Metformin," *New England Journal of Medicine* 346, no. 6 (2002).
34. Ibid.
35. Ibid.
36. Jeffrey A. Katula, Mara Z. Vitolins, Timothy M. Morgan, Michael S. Lawlor, Caroline S. Blackwell, Scott P. Isom, Carolyn F. Pedley, and David C. Goff, "The Healthy Living Partnerships to Prevent Diabetes Study: 2-Year Outcomes of a Randomized Controlled Trial," *American Journal of Preventive Medicine* 44, no. 4, Suppl. 4 (2013).
37. Monika K. Krzyzanowska, R. Kaplan, and Richard Sullivan, "How May Clinical Research Improve Healthcare Outcomes?," *Annals of Oncology* 22, Suppl. 7 (2011).
38. John M. Westfall, James Mold, and Lyle Fagnan, "Practice-Based Research—'Blue Highways' on the NIH Roadmap," *JAMA* 297, no. 4 (2007).
39. Christine Grady, "Ethical Principles in Clinical Research," in *Principles and Practice of Clinical Research*, ed. J. I. Gallin and F. P. Ognibene (San Diego: Academic Press, 2012).
40. "Trials of War Criminals before the Nuremberg Military Tribunals under Control Council Law No. 10" (Washington, DC: U.S. Government Printing Office, 1949).

41. The National Commission for the Protection of Human Subjects of Biomedical and Behavioral Research, "The Belmont Report: Ethical Principles and Guidelines for the Protection of Human Subjects of Research," U.S. Department of Health and Human Services, http://www.hhs.gov/ohrp/humansubjects/guidance/belmont.html.

42. "Code of Federal Regulations," in *45 Public Welfare*, ed. United States Department of Health and Human Services (Washington, DC, 2009).

43. Selina A. Mohammed, Karina L. Walters, June LaMarr, Teresa Evans-Campbell, and Sheryl Fryberg, "Finding Middle Ground: Negotiating University and Tribal Community Interests in Community-Based Participatory Research," *Nursing Inquiry* 19, no. 2 (2012).

44. Karina L. Walters, Antony Stately, Teresa Evans-Campbell, Jane M. Simoni, Bonnie Duran, Katie Schultz, and Deborah Guerrero, "Indigenist Collaborative Research Efforts in Native American Communities," in *The Field Research Survival Guide*, ed. Arlene R. Stiffman (New York: Oxford University Press, 2009).

45. David A. Dzewaltowski, Paul A. Estabrooks, and Russel E. Glasgow, "The Future of Physical Activity Behavior Change Research: What Is Needed to Improve Translation of Research into Health Promotion Practice?," *Exercise and Sport Sciences Reviews* 32, no. 2 (2004).

46. Ibid.

47. Koh et al., "Translating Research Evidence into Practice to Reduce Health Disparities."

48. Mau et al., "Environmental Factors of Obesity in Communities with Native Hawaiians."

49. Nina Wallerstein and Meredith Minkler, *Community-Based Participatory Research for Health* (San Francisco: Jossey-Bass, 2003).

50. Barbara A. Israel, Amy J. Schulz, Edith A. Parker, Adam B. Becker, Alex J. Allen, and Ricardo Guzman, "Critical Issues in Developing and Following Community Based Participatory Research Principles," in *Community-Based Participatory Research for Health*, ed. Meredith Minkler and Nina Wallerstein (San Francisco: Jossey-Bass, 2003).

51. Meredith Minkler and Nina Wallerstein, *Community-Based Participatory Research for Health: From Process to Outcomes* (John Wiley & Sons, 2011).

52. Barbara A. Israel, Amy J. Schulz, Edith A. Parker, and Adam B. Becker, "Review of Community-Based Research: Assessing Partnership Approaches to Improve Public Health," *Annual Review of Public Health* 19, no. 1 (1998).

53. Ibid.

54. Bruce Shiramizu, Cris Milne, Kevin Terada, Kevin Cassel, Rayna K. Matsuno, Jeffery Killeen, Chin-Yuan Liang, Faye Tachibana, Tom Sheeran, James Weihe, and Marc T. Goodman, "A Community-Based Approach to Enhancing Anal Cancer Screening in Hawaii's HIV-Infected Ethnic Minorities," *Journal of AIDS and Clinical Ressearch* 3, no. 6 (2012).

55. Andrea H. Nacapoy, Joseph Keawe'aimoku Kaholokula, Margaret R. West, Adrienne Y. Dillard, Anne Leake, B. Puni Kekauoha, Donna-Marie Palakiko, Andrea Siu, Sean W. Mosier, and Marjorie K. Mau, "Partnerships to Address Obesity Disparities in Hawai'i: The Pili 'Ohana Project," *Hawaii Medical Journal* 67, no. 9 (2008).

56. Israel et al., "Critical Issues in Developing and Following Community Based Participatory Research Principles."

57. Kathryn L. Braun, JoAnn U. Tsark, LorrieAnn Santos, Nia Aitaoto, and Clayton

Chong, "Building Native Hawaiian Capacity in Cancer Research and Programming. A Legacy of 'Imi Hale," *Cancer* 107, no. 8, Suppl. (2006).

58. Joseph K. Kaholokula, Claire K. Townsend, Ka'imi Sinclair, Donna-Marie Palakiko, Emily Makahi, Sheryl R. Yoshimura, JoHsi Wang, Bridget P. Kekauoha, Adrienne Dillard, Cappy Solatorio, Claire Hughes, Shari Gamio, and Marjorie K. Mau, "The Pili 'Ohana Project: A Community-Academic Partnership to Eliminate Obesity Disparities in Native Hawaiian and Pacific Islander Communities," in *Obesity Interventions in Underserved US Communities: Evidence and Directions,* ed. Shiriki K. Kumanyika, Virginia M. Brennan, and Ruth E. Zambrana (Baltimore: Johns Hopkins University Press, 2014).

59. Israel et al., "Critical Issues in Developing and Following Community Based Participatory Research Principles."

60. Ibid.

61. Mele A. Look, Joseph Keawe'aimoku Kaholokula, Amy Carvahlo, Todd B. Seto, and Mapuana de Silva, "Developing a Culturally Based Cardiac Rehabilitation Program: The Hela Study," *Progress in Community Health Partnerships* 6, no. 1 (2012).

62. Israel et al., "Critical Issues in Developing and Following Community Based Participatory Research Principles."

63. Ibid.

64. Shiramizu et al., "A Community-Based Approach to Enhancing Anal Cancer Screening in Hawaii's HIV-Infected Ethnic Minorities."

65. Joseph K. Kaholokula, Rebecca E. Wilson, Claire K. Townsend, Guangxiang Zhang, John Chen, Sheryl R. Yoshimura, Adrienne Dillard, JoHsi W. Yokota, Donna-Marie Palakiko, Shari Gamiao, Claire K. Hughes, Bridget P. Kekauoha, and Marjorie K. Mau, "Translating the Diabetes Prevention Program in Native Hawaiian and Pacific Islander Communities: The Pili 'Ohana Project," *Translational Behavioral Medicine* 4, no. 2 (2014).

66. Ibid.

67. Israel et al., "Critical Issues in Developing and Following Community Based Participatory Research Principles."

68. Kaholokula et al., "The Pili 'Ohana Project."

69. Israel et al., "Critical Issues in Developing and Following Community Based Participatory Research Principles."

70. Braun et al., "Building Native Hawaiian Capacity in Cancer Research and Programming."

71. Shiramizu et al., "A Community-Based Approach to Enhancing Anal Cancer Screening in Hawaii's HIV-Infected Ethnic Minorities."

72. Ibid.

73. Israel et al., "Critical Issues in Developing and Following Community Based Participatory Research Principles."

74. Marguerite J. Ro and Albert K. Yee, "Out of the Shadows: Asian Americans, Native Hawaiians, and Pacific Islanders," *American Journal of Public Health* 100, no. 5 (2010).

75. Mau et al., "Environmental Factors of Obesity in Communities with Native Hawaiians."

76. Braun et al., "Building Native Hawaiian Capacity in Cancer Research and Programming."

77. Israel et al., "Critical Issues in Developing and Following Community Based Participatory Research Principles."

78. Nacapoy et al., "Partnerships to Address Obesity Disparities in Hawai'i."

79. Marjorie K. Mau, Joseph Keawe'aimoku Kaholokula, Margaret R. West, Anne Leake, James T. Efird, Charles Rose, Donna-Marie Palakiko, Sheryl Yoshimura, Puni B. Kekauoha, and Henry Gomes, "Translating Diabetes Prevention into Native Hawaiian and Pacific Islander Communities: The Pili 'Ohana Pilot Project," *Progress in Community Health Partnerships* 4, no. 1 (2010).

80. Ka'imi A. Sinclair, Emily K. Makahi, Cappy Shea-Solatorio, Sheryl R. Yoshimura, Claire K. M. Townsend, and J. Keawe'aimoku Kaholokula, "Outcomes from a Diabetes Self-Management Intervention for Native Hawaiians and Pacific People: Partners in Care," *Annals of Behavioral Medicine* 45, no. 1 (2013).

81. Joseph K. Kaholokula, Bridget P. Kekauoha, Adrienne Dillard, Sheryl R. Yoshimura, Donna-Marie Palakiko, Claire Hughes, and Claire K. Townsend, "The Pili 'Ohana Project: A Community-Academic Partnership to Achieve Metabolic Health Equity in Hawai'i," *Hawaii Journal of Medicine and Public Health* 73, no. 12, Suppl. 3 (2014).

82. Kaholokula et al., "Translating the Diabetes Prevention Program in Native Hawaiian and Pacific Islander Communities."

83. Joseph K. Kaholokula, Claire K. Townsend, Arlene Ige, Ka'imi Sinclair, Marjorie K. Mau, Anne Leake, Donna-Marie Palakiko, Sheryl R. Yoshimura, Bridget P. Kekauoha, and Claire Hughes, "Sociodemographic, Behavioral, and Biological Variables Related to Weight Loss in Native Hawaiians and Other Pacific Islanders," *Obesity* 21, no. 3 (2013).

84. Joseph K. Kaholokula, Marjorie K. Mau, James T. Efird, Anne Leake, Margaret West, Donna-Marie Palakiko, Sheryl R. Yoshimura, Bridget P. Kekauoha, Charles Rose, and Henry Gomes, "A Family and Community Focused Lifestyle Program Prevents Weight Regain in Pacific Islanders: A Pilot Randomized Controlled Trial," *Health Education and Behavior* 39, no. 4 (2012).

85. Israel et al., "Critical Issues in Developing and Following Community Based Participatory Research Principles."

86. Jan Shoultz, Mary Frances Oneha, Lois Magnussen, Mya Moe Hla, Zavi Brees-Saunders, Marissa Dela Cruz, and Margaret Douglas, "Finding Solutions to Challenges Faced in Community-Based Participatory Research between Academic and Community Organizations," *Journal of Interprofessional Care* 20, no. 2 (2006).

87. Kaholokula et al., "The Pili 'Ohana Project."

88. Shiramizu et al., "A Community-Based Approach to Enhancing Anal Cancer Screening in Hawaii's HIV-Infected Ethnic Minorities."

89. Kaholokula et al., "The Pili 'Ohana Project."

90. Jan Shoultz, Lois Magnussen, Karol Richardson, Mary Frances Oneha, Jacquelyn C. Campbell, Doris Segal Matsunaga, Selynda Mori Selifis, Merina Sapolu, Mariama Samifua, Helena Manzano, Cindy Spencer, and Cristina Arias, "Responding to the Needs of Culturally Diverse Women Who Experience Intimate Partner Violence," *Hawaii Medical Journal* 70, no. 1 (2011).

91. David G. Altman, "Sustaining Interventions in Community Systems: On the Relationship between Researchers and Communities," *Health Psychology* 14, no. 6 (1995).

92. John Hatch, Nancy Moss, Ama Saran, Letitia Presley-Cantrell, and C. Mallory, "Community Research: Partnership in Black Communities," *American Journal of Preventive Medicine* 9, no. 6, Suppl. (1993).

93. Athena T. Samaras, Kara Murphy, Narissa J. Nonzee, Richard Endress, Shaneah Taylor, Nadia Hajjar, Rosario Bularzik, Carmi Frankovich, Xin Qi Dong, and Melissa A. Simon, "Community-Campus Partnership in Action: Lessons Learned from the Dupage County Patient Navigation Collaborative," *Progress in Community Health Partnerships* 8, no. 1 (2014).

94. Kaholokula et al., "A Family and Community Focused Lifestyle Program Prevents Weight Regain in Pacific Islanders."

95. Paris Ponder-Brookins, Joyce Witt, John Steward, Douglas Greenwell, Ginger L. Chew, Yvette Samuel, Chinaro Kennedy, and Mary Jean Brown, "Incorporating Community-Based Participatory Research Principles into Environmental Health Research: Challenges and Lessons Learned from a Housing Pilot Study," *Journal of Environmental Health* 76, no. 10 (2014).

96. Syed M. Ahmed, Barbara Beck, Cheryl A. Maurana, and Gail Newton, "Overcoming Barriers to Effective Community-Based Participatory Research in US Medical Schools," *Education for Health: Change in Learning & Practice* 17, no. 2 (2004).

97. Theresa J. Hoeft, Wylie Burke, Scarlett E. Hopkins, Walkie Charles, Susan B. Trinidad, Rosalina D. James, and Bert B. Boyer, "Building Partnerships in Community-Based Participatory Research: Budgetary and Other Cost Considerations," *Health Promotion Practice* 15, no. 2 (2014).

BIBILOGRAPHY

Abraham, Wandersman, and Paul Florin. "Community Interventions and Effective Prevention." *American Psychologist* 58, no. 6–7 (June–July 2003): 441–448.

Ahmed, Syed M., Barbara Beck, Cheryl A. Maurana, and Gail Newton. "Overcoming Barriers to Effective Community-Based Participatory Research in US Medical Schools." *Education for Health: Change in Learning & Practice* 17, no. 2 (2004): 141–151.

Altman, David G. "Sustaining Interventions in Community Systems: On the Relationship between Researchers and Communities." *Health Psychology* 14, no. 6 (November 1995): 526–536.

Balabis, Joseph, Ann Pobutsky, Kathleen K. Baker, Caryn Tottori, and Florentina Salvail. "The Burden of Cardiovascular Disease in Hawaii 2007." Hawaii State Department Health, 2007.

Blaisdell, Richard Kekuni. "Historical and Cultural Aspects of Native Hawaiian Health." *Social Process in Hawaii* 32, no. 1 (1989).

Braun, Kathryn L., JoAnn U. Tsark, LorrieAnn Santos, Nia Aitaoto, and Clayton Chong. "Building Native Hawaiian Capacity in Cancer Research and Programming. A Legacy of 'Imi Hale." *Cancer* 107, no. 8, Suppl. (October 15, 2006): 2082–2090.

"Code of Federal Regulations." In *45 Public Welfare*, ed. U.S. Department of Health and Human Services. Washington, DC, 2009.

Diabetes Prevention Program Research, Group. "Reduction in the Incidence of Type 2 Diabetes with Lifestyle Interventions or Metformin." *New England Journal of Medicine* 346, no. 6 (2002): 393–403.

Dzewaltowski, David A., Paul A. Estabrooks, and Russel E. Glasgow. "The Future of

Physical Activity Behavior Change Research: What Is Needed to Improve Translation of Research into Health Promotion Practice?" *Exercise and Sport Sciences Reviews* 32, no. 2 (April 2004): 57–63.

Earthjustice. "Down to Earth: David Henkin on Oahu's Makua Valley." http://earthjustice.org/features/down-to-earth-david-henkin-on-oahu-s-makua-valley.

Fawcett, Stephen B. "Some Lessons on Community Organization and Change." In *Reflections on Community Organization: Enduring Themes and Critical Issues*, ed. J. Rothman, 314–334. Itasca, IL: F. E. Peacock Publishers, 1999.

Grady, Christine. "Ethical Principles in Clinical Research." In *Principles and Practice of Clinical Research*, ed. J. I. Gallin and F. P. Ognibene. San Diego: Academic Press, 2012.

Hatch, John, Nancy Moss, Ama Saran, Letitia Presley-Cantrell, and C. Mallory. "Community Research: Partnership in Black Communities." *American Journal of Preventive Medicine* 9, no. 6, Suppl. (November–December 1993): 27–34.

"Historical and Cultural Aspects of Native Hawaiian Health: The Health of Native Hawaiians, a Selective Report on Health Status and Health Care in the 1980's." In *Social Process in Hawaii*. Honolulu: University of Hawai'i Press, 1989.

Hoeft, Theresa J., Wylie Burke, Scarlett E. Hopkins, Walkie Charles, Susan B. Trinidad, Rosalina D. James, and Bert B. Boyer. "Building Partnerships in Community-Based Participatory Research: Budgetary and Other Cost Considerations." *Health Promotion Practice* 15, no. 2 (2014): 263–270.

Israel, Barbara A., Amy J. Schulz, Edith A. Parker, and Adam B. Becker. "Review of Community-Based Research: Assessing Partnership Approaches to Improve Public Health." *Annual Review of Public Health* 19, no. 1 (1998): 173–202.

Israel, Barbara A., Amy J. Schulz, Edith A. Parker, Adam B. Becker, Alex J. Allen, and Ricardo Guzman. "Critical Issues in Developing and Following Community Based Participatory Research Principles." In *Community-Based Participatory Research for Health*, ed. Meredith Minkler and Nina Wallerstein , 47–66. San Francisco: Jossey-Bass, 2003.

Kaholokula, Joseph K., Bridget P. Kekauoha, Adrienne Dillard, Sheryl R. Yoshimura, Donna-Marie Palakiko, Claire Hughes, and Claire K. Townsend. "The Pili 'Ohana Project: A Community-Academic Partnership to Achieve Metabolic Health Equity in Hawai'i." *Hawaii Journal of Medicine and Public Health* 73, no. 12, Suppl. 3 (December 2014): 29–33.

Kaholokula, Joseph K., Marjorie K. Mau, James T. Efird, Anne Leake, Margaret West, Donna-Marie Palakiko, Sheryl R. Yoshimura, Bridget P. Kekauoha, Charles Rose, and Henry Gomes. "A Family and Community Focused Lifestyle Program Prevents Weight Regain in Pacific Islanders: A Pilot Randomized Controlled Trial." *Health Education and Behavior* 39, no. 4 (August 2012): 386–395.

Kaholokula, Joseph K., Claire K. Townsend, Arlene Ige, Ka'imi Sinclair, Marjorie K. Mau, Anne Leake, Donna-Marie Palakiko, Sheryl R. Yoshimura, Bridget P. Kekauoha, and Claire Hughes. "Sociodemographic, Behavioral, and Biological Variables Related to Weight Loss in Native Hawaiians and Other Pacific Islanders." *Obesity* 21, no. 3 (March 2013): E196–203.

Kaholokula, Joseph K., Claire K. Townsend, Ka'imi Sinclair, Donna-Marie Palakiko, Emily Makahi, Sheryl R. Yoshimura, JoHsi Wang, Bridget P. Kekauoha, Adrienne Dillard, Cappy Solatorio, Claire Hughes, Shari Gamio, and Marjorie K. Mau. "The Pili 'Ohana Project: A Community-Academic Partnership to Eliminate Obesity Disparities in Native Hawaiian and Pacific Islander Communities." In *Obesity Interventions in Underserved US Communities: Evidence and Directions,* ed. Shiriki K. Kumanyika, Virginia M. Brennan, and Ruth E. Zambrana. Baltimore: Johns Hopkins University Press, 2014.

Kaholokula, Joseph K., Rebecca E. Wilson, Claire K. Townsend, Guangxiang Zhang, John Chen, Sheryl R. Yoshimura, Adrienne Dillard, JoHsi W. Yokota, Donna-Marie Palakiko, Shari Gamiao, Claire K. Hughes, Bridget P. Kekauoha, and Marjorie K. Mau. "Translating the Diabetes Prevention Program in Native Hawaiian and Pacific Islander Communities: The Pili 'Ohana Project." *Translational Behavioral Medicine* 4, no. 2 (June 2014): 149–159.

Kana'iaupuni, Shawn K., Nolan Malone, and Koren Ishibashi. "Ka Huaka'i: 2005 Native Hawaiian Educational Assessment." Honolulu: Kamehameha Schools, Pauahi Publications, 2005.

Katula, Jeffrey A., Mara Z. Vitolins, Timothy M. Morgan, Michael S. Lawlor, Caroline S. Blackwell, Scott P. Isom, Carolyn F. Pedley, and David C. Goff. "The Healthy Living Partnerships to Prevent Diabetes Study: 2-Year Outcomes of a Randomized Controlled Trial." *American Journal of Preventive Medicine* 44, no. 4, Suppl. 4 (April 2013): S324–332.

Koh, Howard K., Sarah C. Oppenheimer, Sarah B. Massin-Short, Karen M. Emmons, Alan C. Geller, and K. Viswanath. "Translating Research Evidence into Practice to Reduce Health Disparities: A Social Determinants Approach." *American Journal of Public Health* 100 Suppl. 1 (April 1 2010): S72–80.

Krzyzanowska, Monika K., R. Kaplan, and Richard Sullivan. "How May Clinical Research Improve Healthcare Outcomes?" *Annals of Oncology* 22, Suppl. 7 (November 2011): vii10–vii15.

Liu, Lihua, Anne-Michelle Noone, Scarlett Lin Gomez, Steve Scoppa, James T. Gibson, Daphne Lichtensztajn, Kari Fish, Lynne R. Wilkens, Marc T. Goodman, Cyllene Morris, Sandy Kwong, Dennis Deapen, and Barry A. Miller. "Cancer Incidence Trends among Native Hawaiians and Other Pacific Islanders in the United States, 1990-2008." *Journal of the National Cancer Institute* 105, no. 15 (August 7, 2013): 1086–1095.

Look, Mele A., Joseph Keawe'aimoku Kaholokula, Amy Carvalho, Todd B. Seto, and Mapuana de Silva. "Developing a Culturally Based Cardiac Rehabilitation Program: The Hela Study." *Progress in Community Health Partnerships* 6, no. 1 (Spring 2012): 103–110.

Look, Mele A., Mililani K. Trask-Batti, Robert Agres, Marjorie L. Mau, and Joseph K. Kaholokula. "Assessment and Priorities for Health & Well-Being in Native Hawaiians & Other Pacific Peoples." Honolulu: Center for Native and Pacific Health Disparaties Research, 2013.

Magnussen, Lois, Jan Shoultz, Karol Richardson, Mary Frances Oneha, Jacquelyn C. Campbell, Doris Segal Matsunaga, Selynda Mori Selifis, Merina Sapolu, Mariama

Samifua, Helena Manzano, Cindy Spencer, and Cristina Arias. "Responding to the Needs of Culturally Diverse Women Who Experience Intimate Partner Violence." *Hawaii Medical Journal* 70, no. 1 (January 2011): 9–15.

Mau, Marjorie K. "Health and Health Care of Native Hawaiian and Other Pacific Islander Older Adults." Retrieved from http://geriatrics.stanford.edu/ethnomed/hawaiian_pacific_islander/. In V. S. Periyakoil, ed., eCampus Geriatrics, Stanford, CA, 2010.

Mau, Marjorie K., Joseph Keawe'aimoku Kaholokula, Margaret R. West, Anne Leake, James T. Efird, Charles Rose, Donna-Marie Palakiko, Sheryl Yoshimura, Puni B. Kekauoha, and Henry Gomes. "Translating Diabetes Prevention into Native Hawaiian and Pacific Islander Communities: The Pili 'Ohana Pilot Project." *Progress in Community Health Partnerships* 4, no. 1 (Spring 2010): 7–16.

Mau, Marjorie K., Kara N. Wong, Jimmy Efird, Margaret West, Erin P. Saito, and Jay Maddock. "Environmental Factors of Obesity in Communities with Native Hawaiians." *Hawaii Medical Journal* 67, no. 9 (2008): 233.

Minkler, Meredith. "Community Organizing Among the Elderly Poor in San Francisco's Tenderloin District." In *Community Organizing and Community Building for Health*, ed. Meredith Minkler, 272–288. New Brunswick, NJ: Rutgers University Press, 2002.

Minkler, Meredith, and Nina Wallerstein. *Community-Based Participatory Research for Health.* San Francisco: Jossey-Bass, 2003.

Mohammed, Selina A., Karina L. Walters, June LaMarr, Teresa Evans-Campbell, and Sheryl Fryberg. "Finding Middle Ground: Negotiating University and Tribal Community Interests in Community-Based Participatory Research." *Nursing Inquiry* 19, no. 2 (June 2012): 116–127.

Nacapoy, Andrea H., Joseph Keawe'aimoku Kaholokula, Margaret R. West, Adrienne Y. Dillard, Anne Leake, B. Puni Kekauoha, Donna-Marie Palakiko, Andrea Siu, Sean W. Mosier, and Marjorie K. Mau. "Partnerships to Address Obesity Disparities in Hawai'i: The Pili 'Ohana Project." *Hawaii Medical Journal* 67, no. 9 (September 2008): 237–241.

The National Commission for the Protection of Human Subjects of Biomedical and Behavioral Research. "The Belmont Report: Ethical Principles and Guidelines for the Protection of Human Subjects of Research." U.S. Department of Health and Human Services, http://www.hhs.gov/ohrp/humansubjects/guidance/belmont.html.

National Institutes of Health. "About NIH." http://www.nih.gov/about/mission.htm.

Naya, Seiji. "Income Distribution and Poverty Alleviation for the Native Hawaiian Community." In *2nd Annual Hawaiian Business Conference.* Honolulu: Office of Hawaiian Affairs, 2007.

Nguyen, Anh Bao, Neetu Chawla, Anne-Michelle Noone, and Shobha Srinivasan. "Disaggregated Data and Beyond: Future Queries in Cancer Control Research." *Cancer Epidemiology Biomarkers and Prevention* 23, no. 11 (November 2014): 2266–2272.

Office of Hawaiian Affairs. "History: The Establishment of OHA." http://www.oha.org/about/history/.

Panapasa, Sela V., Kamana'opono Crabbe, and Joseph Keawe'aimoku Kaholokula. "Efficacy of Federal Data: Revised Office of Management and Budget Standard for Native Hawaiian and Other Pacific Islanders Examined." *AAPI Nexus: Policy, Practice, and Community* 9, no. 1–2 (Fall 2011): 212–220.

Panapasa, Sela V., Marjorie K. Mau, David R. Williams, and James W. McNally. "Mortality Patterns of Native Hawaiians across Their Lifespan: 1990-2000." *American Journal of Public Health* 100, no. 11 (November 2010): 2304–2310.

Pilisuk, Marc, JoAnn McAllister, and Jack Rothman. "Social Change Professionals and Grassroots Organizing : Functions and Dilemmas." In *Community Organizing and Community Building for Health*, ed. Meredith Minkler. New Brunswick, NJ: Rutgers University Press 1997.

Ponder-Brookins, Paris, Joyce Witt, John Steward, Douglas Greenwell, Ginger L. Chew, Yvette Samuel, Chinaro Kennedy, and Mary Jean Brown. "Incorporating Community-Based Participatory Research Principles into Environmental Health Research: Challenges and Lessons Learned from a Housing Pilot Study." *Journal of Environmental Health* 76, no. 10 (June 2014): 8–17.

Protect Kaho'olawe 'Ohana. "History." http://www.protectkahoolaweohana.org.

Ro, Marguerite J., and Albert K. Yee. "Out of the Shadows: Asian Americans, Native Hawaiians, and Pacific Islanders." *American Journal of Public Health* 100, no. 5 (2010): 776–778.

Samaras, Athena T., Kara Murphy, Narissa J. Nonzee, Richard Endress, Shaneah Taylor, Nadia Hajjar, Rosario Bularzik, Carmi Frankovich, XinQi Dong, and Melissa A. Simon. "Community-Campus Partnership in Action: Lessons Learned from the Dupage County Patient Navigation Collaborative." *Progress in Community Health Partnerships* 8, no. 1 (Spring 2014): 75–81.

Shiramizu, Bruce, Cris Milne, Kevin Terada, Kevin Cassel, Rayna K. Matsuno, Jeffery Killeen, Chin-Yuan Liang, Faye Tachibana, Tom Sheeran, James Weihe, and Marc T. Goodman. "A Community-Based Approach to Enhancing Anal Cancer Screening in Hawaii's HIV-Infected Ethnic Minorities." *Journal of AIDS and Clinical Ressearch* 3, no. 6 (August 1, 2012).

Shoultz, Jan, Mary Frances Oneha, Lois Magnussen, Mya Moe Hla, Zavi Brees-Saunders, Marissa Dela Cruz, and Margaret Douglas. "Finding Solutions to Challenges Faced in Community-Based Participatory Research between Academic and Community Organizations." *Journal of Interprofessional Care* 20, no. 2 (2006): 133–144.

Sinclair, Ka'imi A., Emily K. Makahi, Cappy Shea-Solatorio, Sheryl R. Yoshimura, Claire K. M. Townsend, and J. Keawe'aimoku Kaholokula. "Outcomes from a Diabetes Self-Management Intervention for Native Hawaiians and Pacific People: Partners in Care." *Annals of Behavioal Medicine* 45, no. 1 (February 2013): 24–32.

Srinivasan, Shobha, and Tessie Guillermo. "Toward Improved Health: Disaggregating Asian American and Native Hawaiian/Pacific Islander Data." *American Journal of Public Health* 90, no. 11 (November 2000): 1731–1734.

Stafford, Stephen. "Caught between 'the Rock' and a Hard Place: The Native Hawaiian and Pacific Islander Struggle for Identity in Public Health." *American Journal of Public Health* 100, no. 5 (2010): 784–789.

Taualii, Maile, Joey Quenga, Raynald Samoa, Salim Samanani, and Doug Dover. "Liberating Data: Accessing Native Hawaiian and Other Pacific Islander Data from National Data Sets." *AAPI Nexus: Policy, Practice, and Community* 9, no. 1 (2011): 1–7.

"Trials of War Criminals before the Nuremberg Military Tribunals under Control Council Law No. 10," 181–182. Washington, DC: U.S. Government Printing Office, 1949.

"Update on Kanaka Maoli (Indigenous Hawaiian) Health." *Asian American and Pacific Islander Journal of Health* 4, no. 1–3 (Winter 1996): 160–165.

US Census Bureau. "Census Bureau Facts for Features: Asian/Pacific American Heritage Month." https://www.census.gov/newsroom/releases/archives/facts_for_features_special_editions/cb10-ff07.html.

US Congress. "Native Hawaiian Health Care Act of 1988." In *PL 100-579.* Washington, DC, 1988.

U.S. Department of Housing and Urban Development. "Housing Problems and Needs of Native Hawaiians." Washington, DC: U.S. Department of Housing and Urban Development, 1993.

Wagstaff, Adam. "Poverty and Health Sector Inequalities." *Bulletin of the World Health Organization* 80, no. 2 (2002): 97–105.

Walters, Karina L., Antony Stately, Teresa Evans-Campbell, Jane M. Simoni, Bonnie Duran, Katie Schultz, and Deborah Guerrero. "Indigenist Collaborative Research Efforts in Native American Communities." In *The Field Research Survival Guide*, ed. Arlene R. Stiffman, 146–173. New York: Oxford University Press., 2009.

Westfall, John M., James Mold, and Lyle Fagnan. "Practice-Based Research—'Blue Highways' on the NIH Roadmap." *JAMA* 297, no. 4 (January 24, 2007): 403–406.

White House Initiative on Asian Americans and Pacific Islanders. "What You Should Know about Native Hawaiians and Pacific Islanders." Washington, DC: U.S. Department of Education, 2010.

Kalaupapa, a Place Never Forgotten

Kalani Brady and Shelley Soong

"We need Hawaiians taking care of Hawaiians." This statement to me by Dr. Emmett Aluli, a dedicated family practitioner on Moloka'i, explains why Hawaiian physicians—from the State of Hawai'i, through the Department of Native Hawaiian Health at the John A. Burns School of Medicine, University of Hawai'i—took on the honorable role of becoming *nā kauka* (physicians, doctors) for the residents of Kalaupapa. This statement also re-awoke the romantic longing I have held since I was a Hawaiian youth wanting to go into medicine, to be able to spend vast amounts of time with patients. For the State of Hawai'i expects that the duties of *kauka* serving Kalaupapa are not only to meet the medical needs of Kalaupapa residents, but also to spend time with them, listening to their stories. To me, this has never been a "duty" but a gift. The unique opportunity to be a *kauka* in such a special place as Kalaupapa has been a true blessing.

After more than a century of hardships in Kalaupapa, its history shines a bright light on the perseverance of the patients. Their stories have provided a wide range of lessons for the world, such as the vital importance of cultural sensitivity as learned from the failure of a federal research investigation station. Hawaiian values with daily impact are revealed through stories of sacrifice, family, and love. This chapter provides a brief history of Kalaupapa, its current state, valuable lessons learned, and how this special place has provided the world a model of charity, forgiveness, and blessings. This writing is based on numerous readings and reflections, as well as presentations and

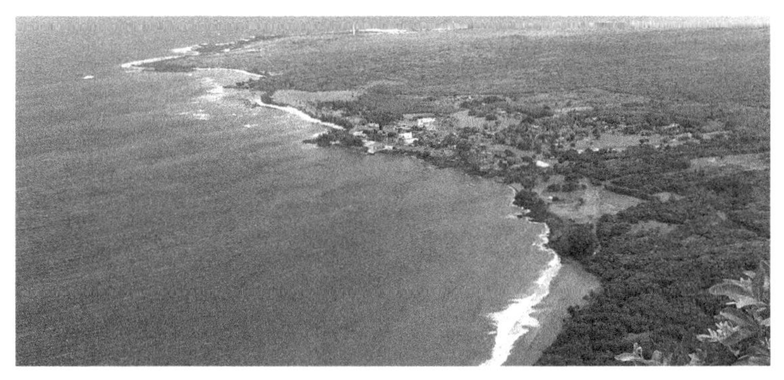

Figure 9.1. Kalaupapa settlement. Photo by Chung-Eun Ha, used with permission.

tours I have given to students, missionaries, and health professionals. It includes viewpoints developed from over a decade in which I have lived, played, and worked with the patients and residents of Kalaupapa.

Hansen's Disease

Hansen's disease is the scientific name of a disease that has been around for thousands of years and is recorded in the Old Testament. It is a chronic infectious disease in the same family of diseases as tuberculosis. The clinical symptoms of Hansen's disease affect mainly the skin and cooler body areas like the upper respiratory tract and testicles. Hansen's disease can also affect areas around the eyes and, before treatment became available, could cause blindness. The nerves can also be affected, and if left untreated, enlargement and malfunction of the peripheral nerves leading to anesthesia (insensitivity to pain or numbness) in the extremities (hands and feet) can lead to amputation of fingers and toes.

Hansen's disease is a communicable disease transmitted in the same way as tuberculosis, by airborne bacteria. In an untreated patient, nasal secretions and the droplets of a cough are loaded with Hansen's disease bacterium; however, unlike tuberculosis, Hansen's disease is not easy to catch. The important point to remember, often not mentioned in historical accounts, is that only 3–5 percent of the world's population is susceptible to Hansen's disease. Is it a pretty rare disease? It is. Yet despite this, worldwide there are still 800,000 new cases each year and as many as two million active Hansen's patients averaging from twenty to thirty years of age. The disease is rare in children younger than five because there is a three- to five-year incubation period, which means once you're exposed to it, and perhaps even exposed to it multiple times, it still takes three to five years for the disease to manifest in clinical situations.

Today in Hawai'i, we catch cases of Hansen's disease in patients as they come into Hawai'i through immigration. We treat them as outpatients, similar to tuberculosis patients. Once treated, patients can't spread the disease and can live in their communities without being at risk to anyone. When Hansen's disease was first introduced to Hawai'i, however, there was no knowledge about treatment, transmission, or the disease itself.

Finding Kalaupapa

In 1778, when Captain James Cook came to Hawai'i, there were 300,000 to 800,000 Native Hawaiians.[1] Over the decades to follow, Western sailors and merchants came to Hawai'i and brought with them the diseases of Europe, the Americas, and Asia. They came with plague, influenza, smallpox, measles, and other diseases that would kill, sometimes, up to a thousand people a day in Hawai'i.[2] Massive disease epidemics decimated the Hawaiian population such that by the mid-nineteenth century, the Hawaiian population plummeted to 30,000.[3] It was a horrific time especially for the ali'i (chiefs) who had to watch their people die.

As this sad and dreadful period for the Hawaiian nation continued, a new disease arrived in the 1840s: Hansen's disease. In a sense, it was worse than other diseases that could kill you in a day. An individual would contract Hansen's disease and suffer for years, progressively looking worse and becoming markedly deformed, eventually dying from the disease in five to seven years. There soon grew a fear that the disease would continue and that Hawai'i would become known as the place of leprosy.

By 1865, King Kamehameha V approved An Act to Prevent the Spread of Leprosy[4] by recommendation of his directors and ministers. This constitutional act mandated that if you were suspected of having Hansen's disease, you were arrested, sent to trial, and if convicted of having the disease, sentenced to imprisonment for life. The Kingdom Board of Health searched for a place to which Hansen's disease patients could be exiled in an attempt to prevent the spread of the disease. Kalaupapa was a large, flat peninsula on the north side of Moloka'i with a long-standing fishing village on the west side but

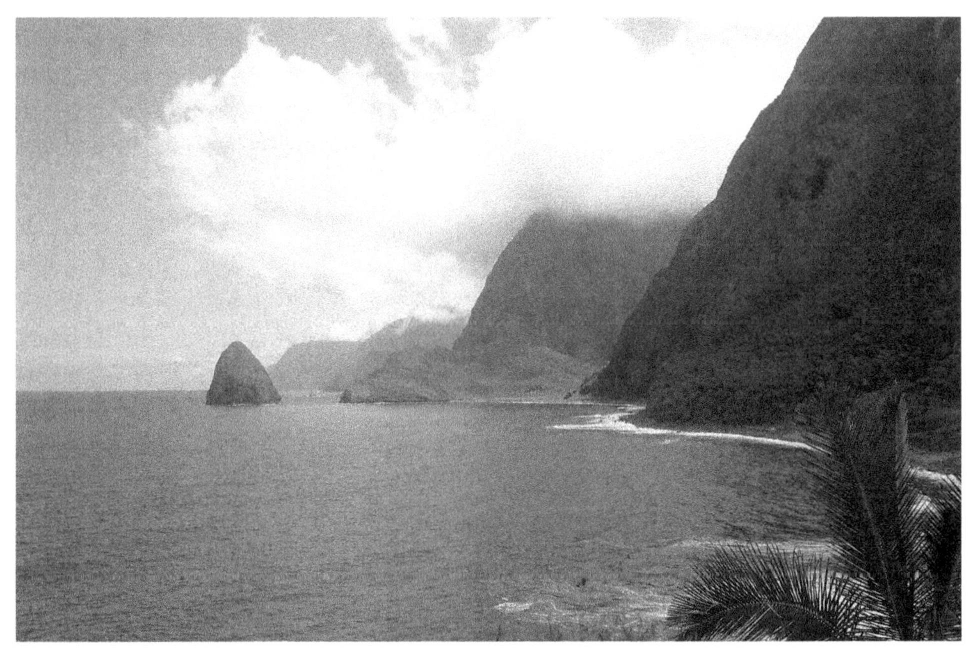

Figure 9.2. Kalawao: Site of the first Hansen's disease settlement. Photo by Chung-Eun Ha, used with permission.

no habitation along the east side, in Kalawao. It was here in Kalawao where the first Hansen's disease settlement was established.[5]

There were several failed attempts to get Hansen's disease patients to the settlement because of weather, landing conditions, and other factors. Also supply ships would leave Honolulu, but never arrive at Kalawao, the untrustworthy captains instead sailing to Tahiti or the Marquesas.[6] Finally, in January of 1866, the first handful, less than a dozen patients, arrived at Kalawao and the Hansen's disease settlement officially came to life.

Imagine having a disease, being arrested for having it, then being exiled for life. That was the fate of those sent to Kalaupapa. Their lives in Kalawao lasted perhaps only five to eight years in which they lived with debilitating disabilities as a result of the disease. As patients watched one another come to the end of their lives, they knew that this would also be their fate. Kalawao became a place of despair. Men were tossed into the settlement and took up with women, girls, and boys, and were basically drunk almost every day. It was a very dark and sinful place.

Saints of Kalaupapa

Saint Damien

Saint Damien was born Jozef de Veuster to a family in Belgium. He came to Hawai'i in 1864 and attended Aliamanu School in Kaneohe on the island of O'ahu. The school grew to what we know today as Saint Louis School, so we have the joy of saying that Saint Damien was, in fact, an alumnus of Saint Louis School! He was later ordained as a Catholic priest at the Cathedral of Our Lady of Peace in Honolulu and took the name Damien. In the 1860s and early 1870s he became an ardent missionary, mostly in Puna and Kohala on the Island of Hawai'i. In 1873 Damien's bishop called him and other missionaries together and told them they had a problem called "Kalawao." The missionaries were told that everyone there was in despair, that there was a lot of darkness with no hope, and there was no one there to teach the people of Kalawao and Kalaupapa the love of God. I imagine Damien would have stepped forward and said, as was written in the biblical scripture Isaiah 6:8: *"Here I am, send me."* It was from here that Damien, pretty much on his own, began his journey of charity and sacrifice first to the people of Kalawao and then as the settlement expanded to Kalaupapa.

When Damien arrived in Kalawao in 1873, there were almost a thousand patients. He quickly started soothing those who were dying. He bandaged their wounds, he built their coffins, and he laid them to rest as they passed. He also took up smoking a pipe because the stench of the patients' sores was so bad. Damien would walk into homes of brigands and remove girls and boys from their illegitimate captivity. He also provided adult women the opportunity to leave the captivity of the brigands, and some would willingly leave to stay with Damien and his growing flock. Eventually, Damien had a group of women, children, and a few men who were at the end of their lives. Together, they celebrated mass, took communion, and administered church sacraments to others.

Damien's selfless service was shared with not only the patients of Kalawao and Kalaupapa, but also others on the island of Moloka'i. The only way out of Kalawao was on foot to Kalaupapa and then up a very steep trail to what patients called the "topside" of Moloka'i. At the top of the trail, however, there was a guard who did not allow the patients through the gate and on to the rest of the island. Damien, however, got through the gate many times and built churches for residents in other parts of Moloka'i, thereby further extending the reach of his selfless service.

One day, after Damien came down the steep trail back to Kalaupapa and then to Kalawao, he decided to soothe his feet in a bucket of warm water. He put one foot in and then the other. Just as the second foot went in he immediately pulled it out because the water was too hot. He knew then that his one foot was numb and that he too had contracted the disease. From then on, he used the language "we lepers" in his sermons.[7] He had become one of them. In the years that followed, he would become not only their priest, but also their community leader. Patients saw Damien as an example because though he was a patient, he still had joy in his heart, and instead of living in despair because of the disease, he lived with joy in the eternal.

He wrote prolifically to the United States and Europe, begging them for support to take care of "his lepers" as he called them. There were times when the bell would toll to announce the passing of a patient as often as two or three times a day. But from the dark state of desolation in which patients had once existed, Damien exacted an overall transformation by way of his care for them.

Saint Marianne

As Damien knew he was dying from Hansen's disease, he asked other religious people to come take care of the patients. Mother Marianne, now known as Saint Marianne, answered a call that Damien had written in a letter to the Order of Saint Francis in Syracuse, New York. When she and two other Franciscan sisters, Leopoldina and Vincentia, first arrived in Hawai'i, they were detained in Honolulu by the prime minister because he felt it was unsafe for them to go to Kalaupapa. In 1888, one year before Damien passed away, they were allowed to begin their service. The sisters set up the Bishop Home with money donated by the Bishop family as the convent and orphanage for girls at Kalaupapa.

Kalaupapa Today

There were seven thousand to eight thousand patients who lived in or passed through Kalawao and Kalaupapa from 1866 to today.[8] Unfortunately, records are incomplete: tsunamis and other natural disasters have displaced graves and decimated graveyards, so it is unknown where all patients are buried, especially those from the early years.

The John A. Burns School of Medicine's Department of Native Hawaiian Health became involved with the patients of Kalaupapa in 2004 when I formed a *hui* (group) of Hawaiian physicians, including Dr. Martina Kamaka, Dr. Peter Donnelly, and later Dr. Chad Koyanagi. We became the doctors that worked with Hansen disease patients, first in Kalaupapa, and later in Honolulu with patients that moved or would leave Kalaupapa for extended periods and live at Hale Mohalu, a part of Lēʻahi Hospital. At the time, there were approximately forty patients in Kalaupapa, all retired, with the youngest about fifty-nine years old. They were still vigorous and enjoyed riding bicycles, playing volleyball, having parties, and playing cards. It was a good time.

Kalaupapa is now a much quieter place. In the twelve years I have been involved, most patients have passed away, and we have just fifteen to sixteen patients between Hale Mohalu and Kalaupapa. Most of those living in Kalaupapa come to Hale Mohalu for special medical visits, such as radiology. In Kalaupapa, most residents prefer to live in their own home. There is a cadre of nurses who care for the patients around the clock. They provide home visits as well as opportunities to go riding and be as comfortable and as joyful as possible. As the years have passed and patient numbers diminished, I became the only doctor who continued to travel regularly to Kalaupapa to provide patient care. The youngest patient is now in their early eighties, and the eldest is ninety. They are very religious as a group, and activities primarily center around church and social events. That is life in Kalaupapa now: very quiet. About forty to fifty state workers help care for patients, and about fifty employees from the National Park Service maintain the historic site of Kalaupapa.

The future of Kalaupapa is somewhat up in the air. The National Park Service has done citizen interviews and community gatherings on all islands to get a sense of what Hawaiʻi's people want for Kalaupapa. In particular, of course, they are interested in what the Hansen's disease patients want for Kalaupapa, and so over the years they have done extensive interviews with the patients. There is a group called Ka ʻOhana O Kalaupapa that is very powerful in determining the future of Kalaupapa. It will probably be a quiet, reflective place where people will come on day trips like they do now. Once the remaining Hansen's disease patients are gone, however, it will be even quieter and hopefully the sacredness of this special place will continue to be felt.

Significant Lessons Learned

Ethical Research

There are important lessons learned from Hansen's disease in Hawai'i that help us remember the history of Kalaupapa. A congressionally authorized U.S. Investigation Station was opened in 1909 at Kalawao and served as a research hospital for Hansen's disease, the first hospital in the United States authorized to research a specific disease. Patients who volunteered to participate in the early research efforts were objectified as "human subjects" for research and were required to live in isolation,[9] banned from contact with family, friends, and anyone outside the Investigation Station. It was closed in 1913 and deemed a failure for reasons including lack of communication between haole scientists and Kalaupapa residents, patients' resentment for their appalling and inhumane incarceration, resentment of the illegal annexation of Hawai'i and takeover of land at Kalawao, and concern that patients were being used as "experimental animals" to learn about the disease to help people beyond Hawai'i.[10] Ruins of the failed station still exist and remain forever a reminder of this valuable lesson.

Cultural Sensitivity

The increase in cultural sensitivity has indeed been a colorful lesson. The word "leprosy" is officially banned in the state of Hawai'i, and patients are referred to as having Hansen's disease to avoid dehumanizing them with the stigma of the term "leprosy." Arresting someone, sending them to trial, convicting them, and then exiling them for a disease, would never occur today. The devil of disease has mauled the physical features of Hansen's disease patients to the point that some of them look disfigured, and for some people that aren't used to relating with people with the disease, they have difficulty seeing Hansen disease patients as people. However, when you get to know the patients beyond physical appearance, you then can genuinely relate lovingly with their heart and soul.

As the Department of Native Hawaiian Health and as a medical school we continually strive to be culturally sensitive. The department does an abundance of community-based participatory research and is considered to be among the leaders in this collaborative research approach.

The Practice of Medicine

When my generation of physicians entered medical practice, it was typical to have extended meaningful interaction with patients. Nowadays doctors are expected to see six to seven patients in an hour, with often less than ten minutes for each patient. As I have practiced over the past thirty years, I have seen medicine taking a turn toward volume-based health care. Physician reimbursements for patient visits now cover just half the amount of what was previously covered when I first began my medical practice, forcing doctors to see many more patients. Being the kauka in Kalaupapa has perhaps given me the opportunity to live my romantic ideal of seeing patients and having them become lifetime friends. My Kalaupapa patients invite me to be the choir director, go bike riding, and be a part of their everyday life. Caring for these patients has been both rewarding and a blessing. We sit and talk about their lives and experiences. The solidarity that exists is very much a positive aspect of the doctor-patient relationship.

There is an immense sadness to Kalaupapa, particularly in what humans did to humans. Medicine, particularly clinical practice, is evolving and changing. Young health practitioners are working in a very different era of health care. It is important to keep the overall tenets the same, that is, to put the patients first, to make sure you enjoy what you're doing in medicine, and to always remember that it is a calling. It is through Kalaupapa that we have had the opportunity to learn these valuable lessons and, even more important, to remember how Kalaupapa has given true meaning to blessings, sacrifice and love.

The authors wish to thank the patients and residents of Kalaupapa. We would also like to thank Mele Look and Lilinoe Andrews, for their assistance in editing; Chung-Eun Ha, for use of his photographs; and The Queen's Health Systems. The content is solely the responsibility of the authors and does not necessarily represent the official views of its funder.

NOTES

1. David E. Stannard, *Before the Horror: The Population of Hawai'i on the Eve of Western Contact* (Honolulu: University of Hawai'i Press, 1989).
2. O. A. Bushnell, *The Gifts of Civilization: Germs and Genocide in Hawai'i* (Honolulu: University of Hawai'i Press, 1993).
3. Ibid.
4. Jerrold M. Michael, "The Public Health Service Leprosy Investigation Station on Molokai, Hawaii, 1909–13—an Opportunity Lost," *Public Health Reports* 95, no. 3 (1980).
5. Gavan Daws, *Holy Man: Father Damien of Molokai* (Honolulu: University of Hawai'i Press, 1973).
6. Ibid.
7. Ibid.
8. Kerri A. Inglis, *Ma'i Lepera* (Honolulu: University of Hawai'i Press, 2013), 196.
9. Ibid.
10. Ibid.

BIBLIOGRAPHY

Bushnell, O. A. *The Gifts of Civilization: Germs and Genocide in Hawai'i.* Honolulu: University of Hawai'i Press, 1993.

Daws, Gavan. *Holy Man: Father Damien of Molokai.* Honolulu: University of Hawai'i Press, 1973.

Inglis, Kerri A. *Ma'i Lepera.* Honolulu: University of Hawai'i Press, 2013.

Michael, Jerrold M. "The Public Health Service Leprosy Investigation Station on Molokai, Hawaii, 1909–13—an Opportunity Lost," *Public Health Reports* 95, no. 3 (1980): 203–209.

Stannard, David E. *Before the Horror: The Population of Hawai'i on the Eve of Western Contact.* Honolulu: University of Hawai'i Press, 1989.

Returning to Health in Hāna, Maui

Diane S. L. Paloma

The enduring personal relationships rooted in the land and built between individuals, families, and community groups are what establish the efficacy and sustainability of Hawaiian health programs.

I first ventured to the remote community of Hāna on the far eastern end of Maui in 1998 to volunteer at a community-based cardiovascular risk clinic that assessed individual, family, and community heart health. It was a health-screening effort designed and tested by a dedicated group of Hawaiian health-care providers on Moloka'i to address the dramatic disparities in rates of heart disease in Native Hawaiians. It was brought to Hāna to reach other isolated rural areas. Then, nearly a decade and a half later, I returned to this ancestral foothold of mine to work on a cardiovascular research grant looking for ways to improve congestive heart failure outcomes for Native Hawaiians. This initiative sought a deeper understanding of causes and solutions to heart health of Kānaka Maoli (Native Hawaiians).

As a descendent of *'ohana* (immediate and extended family) from Ke'anae, a fishing and farming community along the road to Hāna, I seek to fulfill a personal *kuleana* (responsibility) toward the *'āina* (land) of my *kūpuna* (ancestors). My 'ohana farmed the 'āina and my third great-grandfather led the Congregational church there, eventually ending up in Olowalu on the other side of the island. As the current director for Native Hawaiian Health at The Queen's Health Systems, I work toward better health outcomes for Native Hawaiians. This long-standing commitment to Hāna has recently resulted in medical professionals and community members converging to establish sustainable, community-driven activities that will improve health and well-being.

Many factors affect the critical health needs of Native Hawaiians in rural areas: remote locations, limited health services, scarce employment opportunities, and diminished household income. Hāna is a community where resources are constantly needed and access to health care is severely limited. It is federally recognized as a medically underserved area with a significant shortage of health professionals. Without adequate resources to support the health of the community, it is difficult to overcome the dire health statistics of the population. And yet, despite the geographical barriers and persistent challenges that Hāna faces, there are strategies that, when applied, help this community persevere and, we hope, thrive. The most important strategy of all is the formation of personal relationships among those in the community.

The drive to Hāna takes about three hours one way from the Kahului airport and is famous for its hundreds of switchback and hairpin turns, which test my stomach's own strength and persistence every time. The lush beauty and untouched 'āina of Hāna holds a historical reference for Hawaiian history and culture. It is a town isolated by a sixty-four-mile highway with fifty or more one-lane bridges.[1] Ka'uiki Hill in Hāna is the birthplace of noted chiefess Ka'ahumanu, wife of Kamehameha I. Hāna's district has over 60 percent Native Hawaiian residents, one of the highest in the State of Hawai'i.[2] In a time of continual modernization and fast-paced living, Hāna is an example of a true rural community where families depend on each other for all things. It has remained true to its origins as a source of strength and repose, with a fighting spirit for survival. The rain forest and signature Uakea rain shelter the community from the creep of urban infiltration.

The long commute always provides time to prepare for the transformative experiences to come that await among the lush greenery of Hāna's valleys, bays, and rolling hills. I have historical family ties to Hāna, yet I see myself as a visitor on every trip. Each time I have been invited back—invitation to return being the appropriate protocol for entering into Native Hawaiian communities—the beauty has been as breathtaking as ever, but the health needs seem to increase and grow exponentially with each visit.

My first visit to Hāna and the stunning beauty of the 'āina—'Ōhe'o Gulch,

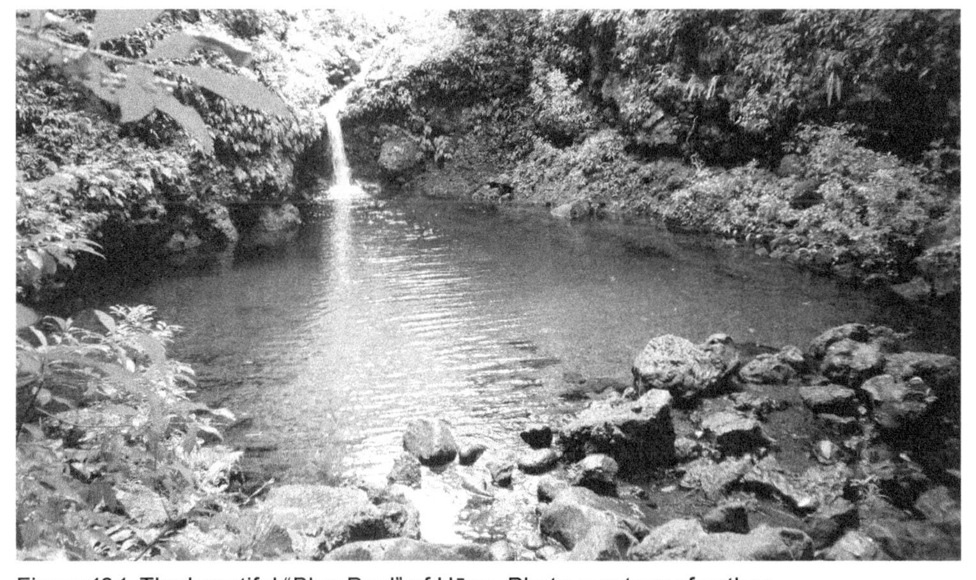

Figure 10.1. The beautiful "Blue Pool" of Hāna. Photo courtesy of author.

Pi'ilani Heiau, and "Blue Pool"—captured my heart and I was never the same. I met community outreach workers that embraced me as a family member, and those relationships became critical to the success of the program. They opened their doors and enabled us to meet others and develop relationships with the larger community. At the time, I didn't really understand why I loved the beauty of the place and the families so much. It was only later that I discovered I had kūpuna who had lived along that same coast and farmed the same land.

In 2012, I reconnected with some old friends. The friendships were picked up where they left off and fostered a trust between those in and beyond the community. The relationships had matured in many ways, and my sense of kuleana was more burdensome than ever because of my role in health care, in light of the dismal reality that the same health conditions we encountered in 1998 seemed to persist with the current generation. Despite advances in health care, Native Hawaiians still were on the unfavorable end of the disparity spectrum.

Each time I left Hāna, whether by car or by plane, I would look back and feel this deep undercurrent of despair and hurt, and those feelings would manifest into my personal commitment to bettering the health of nā po'e Hāna. That feeling created a realization that I have the ability to work in ways that partner with those established relationships. It has strengthened my resolve to brave the long journey to East Maui in order to work there. And it has brought to me a recognition that the needs of Native Hawaiians there are just about the same as their needs in other communities. While working in an office housed in an old-style wooden building, I took the time to walk down the hall and was greeted at each doorway with aloha. The relationships we have built together are what keeps the *pilina* (relationship, union, connection) and strengthens the bonds so much that even after years of distance, friends are still seen as family. This binding of relationships between individuals is the bond that extends far beyond the miles of winding roads and bridges. It is the deep intergenerational bonds that create new 'ohana and ensure connections to the future.

Over the many years of visiting Hāna, I have found a way to maintain a connection to that *wahi pana* (legendary place). Each time, I leave a part of me there to help maintain my connection. By giving of myself to Hāna and its surrounding communities, I feel I am able to receive the spirit of resilience and perseverance. My time there is spent working, but I am able to see and experience what it means to live there. To be included as 'ohana within a community not my own is unique to our experience there. It has also prompted the realization that the strength of Hāna lies in its people. Our work there now is driven by Hāna, and for Hāna. Their understanding and awareness toward improving their own health has transformed their commitment to wellness in perpetuity. The youth are the intergenerational links toward making healthier choices and living those choices daily.

As the Uakea rain clears, each visit reveals something new, and in so many ways provides more healing and realization for me than anything I could contribute. These symbiotic relationships drive and nurture our shared quest for wellness and life.

Mahalo nui loa to The Queen's Health Systems, the Office of Hawaiian Affairs, and participants, staff, friends, and supporters of the Hāna Ola Project.

NOTES

1. "Final Preservation Plan for County of Maui Bridges within the Hāna Highway Historic District," prepared for County of Maui Department of Public Works and Waste Management, 2001, http://www.co.maui.hi.us/DocumentCenter/Home/View/4069.

2. M. A. Look, M. K. Trask-Batti, R. Agres, M. L. Mau, and J. K. Kaholokula, *Assessment and Priorities for Health & Well-Being in Native Hawaiians & Other Pacific Peoples* (Honolulu: Center for Native and Pacific Health Disparities Research, University of Hawai'i, 2013).

Linking Hawaiian Concepts of Health with Epigenetic Research: Implications in Developing Indigenous Scientists

Dana-Lynn T. Ko'omoa and Alika K. Maunakea

The National Institutes of Health (NIH), the largest biomedical research facility in the country, provides infrastructural and funding support to address public health concerns. While there are several, two goals have been recently recognized as major priorities for NIH: 1) to address and reduce diseases of health disparities,[1] and 2) to promote diversity in the biomedical workforce.[2] These goals are inseparable. To seriously address diseases of health disparities in minority and/or indigenous populations, fostering the growth of underrepresented minorities in biomedical research careers is as essential as understanding the molecular etiology of disease. However, in order to engage indigenous populations in the health sciences, career pathway programs that adeptly incorporate cultural concepts of health and wellness with modern approaches in health science are needed. Here, we explore one such link through personal and professional experiences as Hawaiian biomedical researchers in early stage professorships at two indigenous-serving academic institutes in Hawai'i, the University of Hawai'i at Mānoa (UHM) and the University of Hawai'i at Hilo (UHH).

The unique environment within the Department of Native Hawaiian Health (DNHH) at the John A. Burns School of Medicine in UHM offers an opportunity for basic biomedical researchers to collaborate with a cadre of clinical, behavioral, and health disparities' researchers. DNHH is the only medical school department in the country focused on health disparities of Indigenous Peoples. Health disparities include diseases for which there is clearly a higher prevalence in one particular population—this includes chronic disorders, where there has typically been a large clinical focus. However, the DNHH uses a multidisciplinary approach, which includes basic science perspectives, to address these clinical problems. The integration of several fields of health sciences is important to address health disparities in Hawaiian and Pacific Islander communities because the origin of such health issues are complex and multivariate. In addition, an integrative approach is compatible with the holistic view of health and wellness embedded in traditional Hawaiian culture, called *mauli ola*.[3]

Nā honua mauli ola[4] is a Hawaiian philosophy of health that encompasses the understanding that health (*mauli ola*) is connected and central to three core elements of the human experience, the *piko*: *'ī* (spiritual connection), *'ō* (inherited connection), and *'ā* (the creative/procreative connection). These *piko*[5] connections operate within three environments (*honua*)—family, community, and nation/world—which are experienced over an individual's life span from childhood (*keiki*) to adulthood (*mākua*) to elder (*kūpuna*) status.[6] Disruption of any one of the *piko* connections during any phase of development is thought to cause imbalance of *mauli ola* and lead to health problems.

To enrich and maintain a balance of all three *piko* connections essential for good health, traditional Hawaiian principles and practices were indoctrinated into society. Principles such as *aloha*,[7] *lōkahi*,[8] and *laulima*[9] and practices such as *mālama 'āina*,[10] *ho'oponopono*,[11] and *lā'au lapa'au*[12] are manifestations of *nā honua mauli ola* philosophy. An important aspect central to this philosophy is the interconnectedness of the environment and health. This could include social environment to mental/emotional/spiritual health, as evidenced by practices of *ho'oponopono* or physical environment to physical health as evidenced by practices of *mālama 'āina* or *lā'au lapa'au*. Engaging in these practices reinforce the principles essential to living a balanced lifestyle within the framework of *nā honua mauli ola*. Perturbations in this balance mediated by drastic changes in the environment result in cultural trauma for Indigenous Peoples post-"Western" colonization. This extrinsically induced imbalance of *mauli ola* may underlie the increased burden of chronic disease conditions Hawaiians and Pacific Islanders experience today.

Role of the Environment on Diseases of Health Disparities

According to a report released in 2013 by the DNHH, "In general, Hawaiians and Pacific Islanders (NHPI) bear a disproportionately higher prevalence of many chronic medical conditions, such as obesity, diabetes, and cardiovascular disease, collectively known as cardiometabolic disorders. . . . Hawaiians not only have higher rates of death for diabetes and heart disease but also for cancer and other leading causes of death as compared to the overall State's population."[13] Although these diseases arise under specific genetic circumstances, DNA sequence alone does not fully explain their origin. Indeed, the diseases of health disparities likely originate from a combination of gene-environment interactions, consistent with the Hawaiian concept of mauli ola. The model that best characterizes this critical interface is centered in the study of epigenetics.

Briefly, studies of epigenetics attempt to understand cell intrinsic and extrinsic interactions involved in modulating chromatin to influence gene transcription and other important cellular activities without inducing changes to DNA sequence, and heritably, but reversibly, modifying cell and organismal phenotypes. For example, behavioral and environmental factors such as stress and diet impact the "epigenome" and can lead to heightened risk for and development of disease without alterations to DNA sequence. In cancer, for instance, epigenetic alterations often precede genetic abnormalities, that later intensify tumor progression.[14] Although incompletely understood, dietary nutrients such as folate play important roles during early fetal development and even adulthood in establishing and maintaining normal cell epigenomes because they supply essential metabolites to ensure the proper function of epigenetic regulators.[15] Several studies have revealed that the maternal environment can condition the health of the offspring through epigenetic patterning, which may also have an impact on the health of future generations.[16] By scanning for epigenetically labile sites within the genome that become altered early in disease progression and by identifying cell extrinsic or environmental factors that predispose to disease, diagnostic and preventive strategies can be developed. Thus, epigenetics provides an important and tractable model of gene-environment interactions that are thought to be critical in the development of diseases of health disparity and offers new opportunities for intervention. In the etiology of developmental and chronic diseases, inflammatory pathways regulated by the epigenetic process are conditioned by environmental factors associated with lifestyle. Understanding these associations and restoring a healthier lifestyle may reverse deleterious epigenetic patterns that influence cell function and reduce disease incidence and/or prevent disease progression. This provides a working model with which to study the impact of environment on health.

Chronic inflammation appears to be a common feature of diseases such as heart disease, diabetes, neurological disorders, and cancer (see Figure 11.1). Epigenetic processes may be modified by environmental factors that relate to lifestyle, including diet and behavior, which may impact how certain immune cells are regulated and interact with the gut microbiota. Cellular stressors such as toxicants, stress, free radicals, and others that can be derived from environmental sources may lead to chronic inflammatory states via modifying epigenetic processes, which over time could lead to disease progression. Deleterious, or disease-related, epigenetic changes can be reversed and lead to reduced inflammatory states of immune cells upon engaging in healthier lifestyles including regular exercise, stress management, improved nutrition, etc.[17]

Within the context of "environment," Hawaiians and other Indigenous

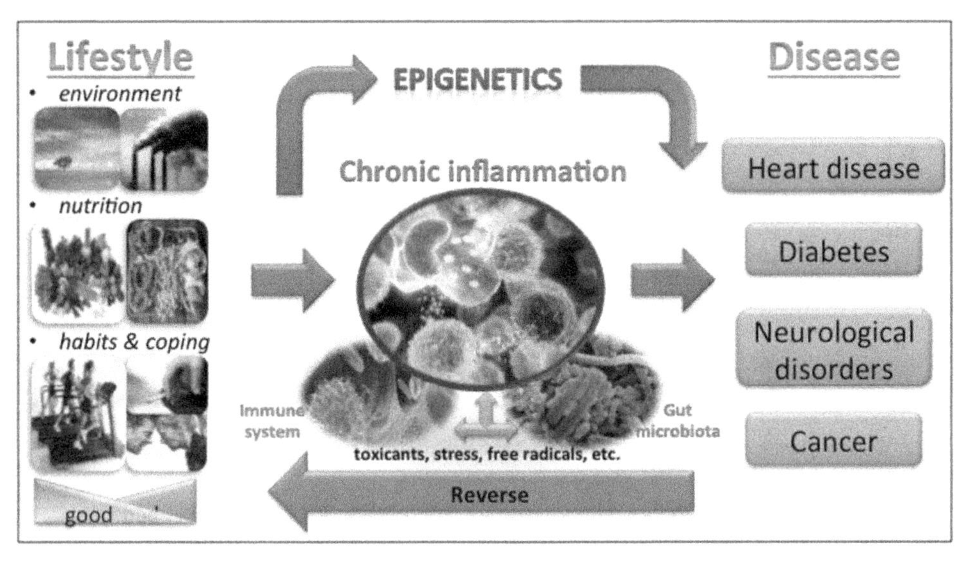

Figure 11.1. Epigenetic processes may mediate the link between lifestyle and disease outcomes.

Peoples experience low educational attainment, poor social-economic status, political disempowerment, ecological and environmental injustices, disenfranchised communities, and cultural loss, all of which contributes to poor dietary decisions, imbalanced nutrition, emotional and physical stress, drug and alcohol abuse, and behavioral problems. Any combination of these social determinants of health, which relate to cultural trauma, may underlie the increased prevalence of chronic diseases observed in Hawaiian and indigenous populations. Understanding how these extrinsic factors affect the epigenome will not only lead to new ways to eliminate diseases of health disparity in Hawaiian and Indigenous Peoples, but may also be applicable to other populations worldwide affected by similar social-environmental circumstances. There is evidence that exposure to these environments may have transgenerational impact on health, through epigenetic mechanisms.[18] Therefore, ongoing behavioral, clinical, and epigenetic studies facilitated through the Department of Native Hawaiian Health applies an integrated approach toward health disparities' research, while incorporating Hawaiian perspectives of health and wellness.

Understanding that the environment, whether social or physical, plays an important role in health was so essential to Hawaiians that ʻōlelo noʻeau[19] abound illustrating this concept in day-to-day practice. As an example *"Pūʻali kalo i ka wai ʻole,"*[20] meaning "Taro, for lack of water, grows misshapen," suggests that lack of caring for the land leads to illness. Another example, *"I paʻa ke kino o ke keiki i ka lāʻau,"* meaning "that the body of the child be solidly built by the medicines," was said of mothers eating herbs (dietary supplements) prescribed by lāʻau lapaʻau practitioners during pregnancy and nursing for the sake of the baby's health during development, as well as to aid in prevention of adult-onset diseases. By conditioning the prenatal environment with medicinal herbs, Hawaiians were shaping the epigenetic patterns of their children with the notion of strengthening their health throughout their life span and into the next generation. These ʻōlelo noʻeau express a fundamental idea of mauli ola in the traditional Hawaiian perspective of wellness, compatible with epigenetics. Indeed, we recently discovered that the natural products used in Hawaiian medicine may operate through epigenetic mechanisms.[21] These results suggest that traditional Hawaiian concepts of wellness included a mechanistic understanding for the role of the environment on physical health—a notion we now recognize as epigenetics.

Due to the compatibility of Hawaiian concepts of health and wellness with the epigenetic etiology of disease, the Maunakea lab incorporates *ʻike kūpuna* in biomedical research activities, including recruiting and engaging the Hawaiian and Pacific Islander community as participants or students in research (see Figure 11.2). Using a multidisciplinary approach to include basic science (in this case epigenetics), clinical research, behavioral medicine, and opportunities for community engagement, we address a variety of diseases facing our society such as neurodevelopmental disorders, cardiometabolic diseases, and cancer. Examples of each appear under each category. By incorporating both a

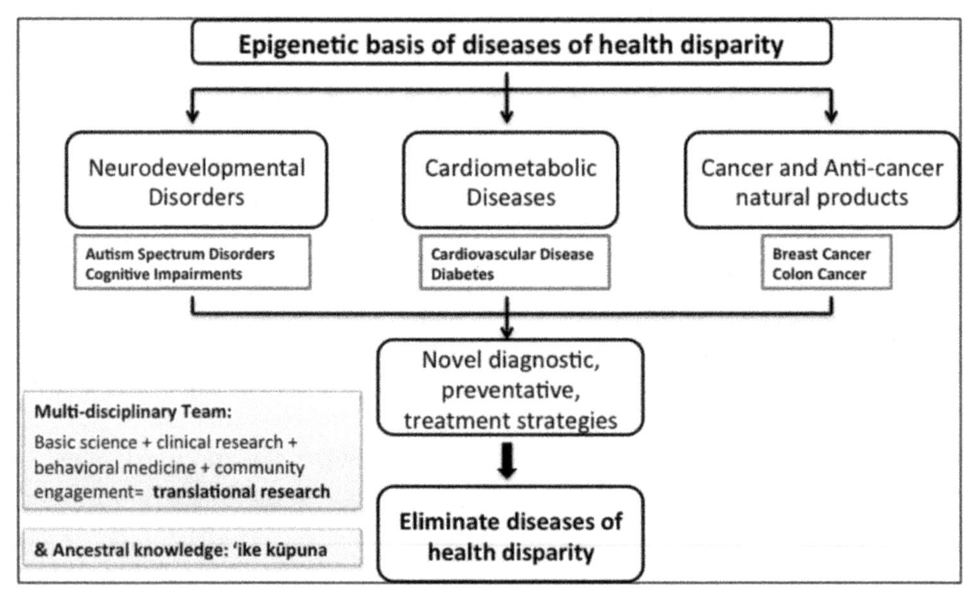

Figure 11.2. Ongoing studies in the Maunakea lab focus on the epigenetic basis of diseases of health disparity.

biomedical strategy of research (i.e., multidisciplinary approach in epigenetics) with ancestral knowledge (*'ike kūpuna*) and cultural perspectives (i.e., *mauli ola*), novel diagnostic, preventative, and treatment strategies could be developed to eliminate these diseases of health disparities in indigenous populations.

Culturally Inspired Research in Health Science Career Pathways

Research that incorporates 'ike kūpuna with modern scientific tools may lead to the development of positive solutions that address diseases of health disparity in a culturally relevant context. In the Maunakea lab, we incorporate such 'ike in understanding the epigenetic basis of diseases of health disparity. (See graphic above.) By doing so, we hope to provide promising solutions to the health challenges that our community (*lāhui*) encounters today, for a better future. Engaging Hawaiian and Pacific Islander students in health science career pathways reinforces this culturally inspired approach to research and provides a way to sustain such studies for future generations. However, in order to provide a sustainable pathway for students to succeed in a biomedical research career, there are other aspects of academic training that should also be addressed. These are highlighted below.

Developing a Health Disparities' Research Workforce

In collaboration with leading members of community-engaged research and education, we propose a potential sustainable pathway for future students to pursue biomedical research in Hawai'i. Some key recommendations for a successful pathway program for students to pursue a biomedical research career include providing: 1) a solid foundation in the sciences, 2) effective mentorship, 3) opportunities for students to engage with their communities during the course of the research, and 4) hands-on real-world experience. While this is by no means an exhaustive list, we highlight these four recommendations and offer our perspective on each.

While many programs can facilitate training students interested in biomedical research careers, few incorporate an indigenous perspective into the training process (see Figure 11.3). In order to seriously address the low numbers of academic research professionals from Hawaiian and Pacific Islander backgrounds, there are four fundamental areas in the training process where both the education in and engagement of the research should incorporate a perspective relevant to Hawaiians and Pacific Islanders, listed here and further explained below. Doing so would yield successful holistic Hawaiian and Pacific Islander biomedical researchers with an intrinsically vested interest in

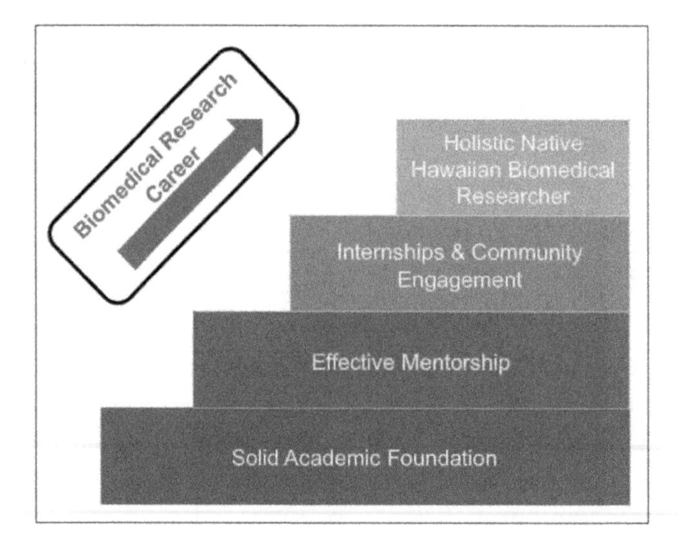

Figure 11.3. An indigenous pathway toward a biomedical research career.

giving back to their community and improving health. Although this pathway is by no means a definitive strategy, it provides a basic guiding principle for biomedical research programs serving indigenous students. As such, we anticipate that while the principles may be fundamental, the specific research activities and how they are delivered to and incorporate students and their communities will inevitably evolve over time.

Recommendation 1: Solid Academic Foundation

I pa'a ke kāhua a laila hiki ke kūkulu
When the foundation is solid only then can you build

A pathway program dedicated to increasing diversity in the health science research workforce in Hawai'i should focus on helping students to acquire the skills and knowledge to obtain and enjoy a successful and rewarding career in biomedical research. Students should obtain skills that will help them to learn and retain knowledge from relevant science courses (e.g., math, chemistry, and biology), and successfully complete coursework to continue advancing in the biomedical sciences program. Many students, particularly Hawaiian and Pacific Islander students, come from cultures that are still largely based on a strong oral tradition, and they still value personal connection. Consequently, students typically perform better with group activities. Consistent with nā honua mauli ola concepts for education, a pathway program should foster an environment that promotes group study in order to achieve academic excellence individually and collectively in the classroom among peers.[22] Peers can provide tutoring, advice, and clarification of scientific concepts. Having good study habits and time management and a network of supportive colleagues creates a solid foundation that is associated with science research careers. Providing a group learning experience will also build camaraderie and help students achieve a sense of belonging, in addition to developing critical social and collaborative skills needed in multidisciplinary health sciences.

In Hawaiian culture, leadership roles are based on *kuleana* (responsibility). There is the *kumu* (teacher), *alaka'i* (leader of the students), and *haumāna* (students). There are instances in which alaka'i take on some teaching and mentoring responsibilities for the kumu and work directly with other students. This allows the alaka'i to obtain training to eventually become a kumu, and it allows haumāna to learn from peers. Often, NHPI students are more comfortable directing questions to a peer rather than a professor. Therefore, learning in a group environment provides more opportunities for these students to develop a strong science background on which to build a career in biomedical science research, and to train more experienced students to take on leadership and mentoring roles. The Native Hawaiian Science and Engineering Mentorship Program (NHSEMP) and Native Hawaiian Student Services (NHSS) offered at the University of Hawai'i at Mānoa provide such support.

Pursuing a degree in biomedical sciences is technically difficult and requires dedication and perseverance to learn a large amount of material and to apply the knowledge to biomedical research. In addition to this, however, Hawaiian and Pacific Islander students face profound cultural obstacles in academia. The obstacles that these students face as undergraduate and graduate students are not only the obvious ones such as the large amount of material they need to learn, progressing in research projects, and economic hardship or lack of educational resources. NHPI students face less apparent but equally important obstacles as well. For instance, NHPI students often need to learn how to present themselves in a professional manner, present their work, and communicate and network with professors and peers, most of whom are from different cultures. Many NHPI students feel uncomfortable with this aspect of their training as the ways of communicating and interacting that are prized in academia and industry—self-assurance while presenting, taking credit for and discussing one's own accomplishments—appear as superiority, arrogance, and overconfidence in Hawaiian culture, where deference and humility are prized. These cultural considerations create obstacles for NHPI students wishing to enter and succeed in a career in biomedical sciences. Therefore, programs should include activities to empower these students and to help them build a strong foundation that also addresses these aspects of their training. The heritage of Hawai'i reflects the rich mix of Hawaiians, Asia-Pacific Islanders, local, national, and international cultures. Therefore, fostering cultural awareness will help to promote an intellectual and social environment for students to learn, practice, and hone critical professional communication skills in a safe setting so that they may develop these skills while maintaining a strong sense of self and following his or her cultural traditions. By creating a learning environment that is conducive to educational effectiveness for students from diverse backgrounds, this program will also prepare students for effective engagement and leadership in biomedical sciences.

Recommendation 2: Effective Mentorship

Nā Pouhana
People on whom you depend for leadership, guidance, and help

Mentors are essential for a successful career in health sciences. They can come in all forms. They should be someone who provides support, whether emotional or academic. Students will obtain relevant and effective mentorship that includes at least three different mentors including, but not limited to, a peer mentor, an emotional mentor, and a professional mentor. Peer-to-peer mentoring enables students to confide in each other and get helpful tips on things such as professors' personalities and teaching styles, homework assignments, writing, and even good free meals. An emotional mentor helps maintain work-life balance by providing support when facing personal problems that could interfere with productivity. Professional mentors have experience in the science field and create opportunities for young researchers to explore possible career paths.

There are many different ways that programs create mentorship opportunities. The most common is a natural professional mentorship that occurs through a training internship program. While professional mentorships may be crucial for providing support and guidance through the degree program and upon entering a career path, it does not always provide support in other critical areas such as emotional mentorship. Other networks are also available through distance learning online.

Hawaiian culture has a heavy emphasis on balance. Being a Hawaiian or Pacific Islander and a scientist is an incredibly delicate negotiation between two worlds with different cultural and social expectations. In NHPI cultures, the family and community are priorities, and NHPIs work toward maintaining and/or improving both. Professional mentors do not always understand other cultures or they believe that cultural considerations should be excluded from professional matters. This lack of emotional support and guidance leaves students with the mistaken impression that in order to succeed, they need to "fit into the system" and *only* focus on building skill sets that are prized by accomplished professors at U.S. academic institutions. Due to the absence of appropriate role models and mentors for NHPI students who understand the challenges and unique perspectives of underrepresented minority scientists, NHPI students continue to struggle in biomedical degree programs and careers. All students need emotional support and guidance. Some students need emotional mentors who will understand that the challenges and unique perspectives of underrepresented minorities are in fact an asset, that these differences constitute a diversity that is important to enhance research. These emotional mentors support students as they develop and cultivate better and unique research ideas and approaches afforded by their ethnic and cultural backgrounds. In this aspect of mentorship, personal relationship is a key component to identifying an advisor who supports not only academic development but personal development, and will be critical to the student's success. Multiple mentors, whether or not in the same department or research division, interact and cooperate to support the student and implement a coordinated plan for career development, personal growth, and achievement.

Mentorship is crucial to maintaining progress in any pathway to success. However, fostering relationships between students and mentors can prove to be quite difficult, especially when there are no definitive guidelines. There should be a general outline of expectations for the mentor-mentee relationship that includes goals and outcomes. At the 2014 Minority Health and Health Disparities conference, many of the professionals that serve as mentors requested that mentees be passionate, humble, and honest. Some good traits to look for in a mentor are someone who is available, respected in their field, successful in life, and whose life students can envision as their own future.[23]

Recommendation 3: Internships and Community Engagement

Ho'i hou i ka mole
Give back to the ancestral root, the community

Identifying research relevance with community values/perspectives is important for engaging NHPI students in health sciences. MA'O Organic Farms executive director Kukui Maunakea-Forth understands the importance of connecting community and research. MA'O has developed a Youth Leadership Training (YLT) where students gain work and leadership experience through "edu-preneurial" internship opportunities with community and academic organizations. Recently, MA'O partnered with the University of Hawai'i's Department of Native Hawaiian Health to administer the Partnership for Improving Lifestyles Intervention (PILI) program, a community-based research program that addresses obesity and related disparities in

Hawai'i. One of the YLT student interns expressed how the PILI internship influenced their future goals and aspirations:

> When conducting any kind of research within a community such as Wai'anae, it is my belief that the best way to get any type of substantial feedback and results is to utilize the community itself rather than bringing in outside specialists. No one knows the community better than those who live in it. The fact that we utilized young adults who are community members was by far the most enjoyable part of the Project. Working in my community alongside these young adults is just amazing. MA'O YLT intern, 2015

From the PILI project student interns learned key concepts, tools, and processes, and developed community-based participatory research skills that were significant in increasing knowledge, integrating the knowledge, and transforming it into interventions and policy that improves the health and well-being of their community.

The expansive community provides the reason for research. Often results generated by biomedical research are presented in a scientific forum that limits the accessibility of research for their community. Pathway programs for future biomedical researchers should partner with the community to create an immediate relationship between the research and the people most affected by their research in order to better understand the needs of the community, as demonstrated by MA'O, because ultimately results generated by biomedical researchers can be of tremendous value to the community. In addition, when students connect and/or find their research relevant to the community, they are more invested in the project. Researchers could also play an important role in inspiring students from the community in which the study is based, recruiting them for future careers in health sciences.

In addition to serving community, place-based learning and *huaka'i* (field trips) to *wahi pana* (legendary, famous sites) provide unique opportunities for students to feel an organic connection to the places and communities they work with. The place/environment cultivates a strong sense of kuleana to NHPI students, since these places serve as physical connections to their ancestry and culture. The research projects, in addition to being in line with students' interest, serve as a vehicle to improve the health and well-being of a community, and the success of the community means a successful project. Rather than being project-centric and self-serving, the kuleana of the student will foster respect for the place and the community. Through mutual respect, the student may develop collaborations with the community and work together to improve the health and well-being of that community. Hawaiian values and perspectives are key components to a successful community service project.

Recommendation 4: Real-World Training Experience

Ma ka hana ka ʻike
In work there is knowledge

Motivation and dedication are needed to succeed in a health science research career. Working in a field that allows students to engage in community-relevant research is one way to maintain these values. Kamehameha Schools–Kapālama has developed two programs, the Kamehameha Summer Science Institute (KSSI) and the Kamehameha Honors Science Research (HSR) program, designed for students to gain hands-on experience in a molecular and cell biology laboratory, learning techniques that are used in both academic and industrial biomedical research careers and have attracted student participation by creating an engaging, exciting environment with hands-on and community-based activities. Alumni of the KSSI and HSR programs have been very successful in health science careers. As a biology teacher with tweny-four years of experience with KSSI and HSR programs, Ms. Gail Ishimoto states:

> Part of the success of KSSI and HSR is that students are encouraged to explore their own interests, using molecular tools. When students have the freedom to explore their own interests, they are empowered and take ownership of their projects. Their first year in KSSI/HSR often leads to summer research internships in university laboratories locally and on the mainland.[24]

Hawaiian and Pacific Islander students traditionally learn through observation and guided practice. NHPI students perform better in an applied learning environment than in a Western learning environment, and benefit from one-on-one contact with teachers to apply what is learned in the classroom to research. Therefore, applied learning experiences for NHPI students, like KSSI/HSR, provide guidance and support to prepare NHPIs to thrive in degree programs and careers in biomedical sciences. Internships are an effective pedagogical tool to enhance the academic experience of NHPI students.

Internships play a major part in a pathway to science research careers because they are a great way for students to learn more about the various fields of biomedical research by doing rather than reading from a textbook. Internships allow students to experience and see the work that is done in biomedical research, physically. During internships, students are exposed to a possible career path early. Internships can also lay the foundation for students and organizations to contribute to meaningful and relevant research through authentic engagement with the community. Partnering with local community organizations can aid with providing internship opportunities for students interested in biomedical research. Having the "buy-in" from the community may also help to maintain a sustainable source of funding for a potential biomedical research pathway that can directly affect their community. Having the community workforce included in the pathway will help foster future generations of scientific researchers.

Furthermore, providing opportunities for culturally inspired research will further engage NHPI students in biomedical research. When there is a cultural component that students can relate to, they become more engaged in learning. The students view the work positively, and they are motivated and inspired by the work. This type of research experience can provide the spark for some students to become interested in biomedical research, or cultivate the curiosity and drive of students who are already interested in pursuing a career in biomedical sciences.

Summary

Hawaiians, Pacific Islanders, Native Americans, and Native Alaskans make up less than 2.5 percent of STEM majors. Fewer than one hundred Hawaiians have a PhD in science. The shortage of NHPIs in biomedical sciences plays a contributory role in health disparities among Hawaiian and Pacific Islanders. Therefore, we need to strengthen the science research workforce in Hawai'i in order to foster more relevant science to investigate disparities in local communities that continue to disproportionately affect these populations.

A sustainable pathway for future researchers needs to be established in order to produce more biomedical researchers in Hawai'i with a solid understanding of indigenous values, practices, and behaviors, so they can implement them in their scientific research careers. Obstacles include limited funding for educational support services and difficulties in establishing sustainable programs that provide quality mentorship and internship opportunities that engage students in research. To overcome these obstacles, we propose a sustainable pathway program that will: 1) provide the resources and opportunities for students to build a solid foundation in sciences in order to thrive in a degree program and career in biomedical sciences, 2) provide the infrastructure for strong mentor-mentee relationships, 3) develop research projects that engage the community, and 4) allow students the opportunity to gain hands-on experience through internships. This sustainable pathway will foster the growth of underrepresented minorities in biomedical research careers, which in turn will address diseases of health disparity in minority and/or indigenous populations.

We wish to thank *(mahalo)* Kelsea Hosoda, a 2015 MS graduate of the Molecular Biosciences and Bioengineering Program at UH Mānoa from the Maunakea lab, whose experience as a Hawaiian student in biomedical research inspired this article. We also would like to mahalo Annette Lum-Jones of the Maunakea lab, who helped with organization and revisions to this work. We send a special mahalo nui loa to Mrs. Kukui Maunakea-Forth of MA'O Organic Farms (Wai'anae, O'ahu), Ms. Gail Ishimoto of Kamehameha Schools (Kapālama, O'ahu), Mrs. Gail Makuakāne-Lundin (UH Hilo), and Taupouri Tangarō (Hawai'i Community College) for sharing valuable knowledge and experience *(mana'o)* that enabled this work.

NOTES

1. See http://www.nimhd.nih.gov/about/vision-mission.html for further information.
2. See http://commonfund.nih.gov/diversity/ for further information.
3. *Mauli ola,* traditional Hawaiian culture.
4. Concepts are elaborated extensively in Native Hawaiian Education Council and UH Hilo in *Na Honua Mauli Ola: Hawaii Guidelines for Culturally Responsive Learning Environments* (Hilo: UH-Hilo 2002).
5. When used in this context, *piko* refers to a connection.
6. Native Hawaiian Education Council.
7. *Aloha,* love, compassion, kindness, sympathy.
8. *Lōkahi,* unity, harmony, accord.
9. *Laulima,* cooperation.
10. *Mālama 'āina,* take care or preserve the land.
11. *Ho'oponopono,* to be correct.
12. *Lā'au lapa'au,* medicine.
13. Mele A. Look et al., "Health Disparities and Health Care Services," in *Assessment and Priorities for Health and Well-Being in Native Hawaiians and Other Pacific Peoples* (Honolulu: University of Hawai'i, 2013).
14. Hong et al., "Shared Epigenetic Mechanisms in Human and Mouse Gliomas Inactivate Expression of the Growth Suppressor SLC5A8," *Cancer Research* 65, no. 9 (2005).
15. Maunakea, Chepelev, and Zhao, "Epigenome Mapping in Normal and Disease States," *Circ Res* 107, no. 3 (2010).
16. Ibid.
17. Unpublished observation by A. K. Maunakea.
18. Maunakea et al.
19. *'Ōlelo no'eau,* proverb.

20. Quoted from M. K. Pukui, *'Ōlelo No'eau: Hawaiian Proverbs and Poetical Sayings* (Honolulu: Bishop Museum Press, 1983).

21. Ka'ahukane Leite-Ah Yo, "E hō mai ka 'ike kūpuna no ke ola: Links between Traditional Native Hawaiian Concepts of Health and Epigenetic Research," *Hulili,* under review, 2015.

22. Native Hawaiian Education Council.

23. A good resource can be found at National Institute of Health: www.training.nih.gov/mentoring_guidelines.

24. Gail Ishimoto, KHS, 2015.

BIBLIOGRAPHY

Ching, T. T., A. K. Maunakea, P. Jun, C. Hong, G. Zardo, D. Pinkel, J. F. Costello, et al. "Epigenome Analyses Using BAC Microarrays Identify Evolutionary Conservation of Tissue-Specific Methylation of SHANK3." *Nature Genetics* 37, no. 6 (2005): 645–651. doi: 10.1038/ng1563.

Corley, M. J., W. Zhang, X. Zheng, A. Lum-Jones, and A. K. Maunakea. "Semiconductor-Based Sequencing of Genome-Wide DNA Methylation States." *Epigenetics* 10, no. 2 (2015): 153–166. doi: 10.1080/15592294.2014.1003747.

Hong, C., A. Maunakea, P. Jun, A. W. Bollen, J. G. Hodgson, D. D. Goldenberg, J. F. Costello, et al. "Shared Epigenetic Mechanisms in Human and Mouse Gliomas Inactivate Expression of the Growth Suppressor SLC5A8." *Cancer Research* 65, no. 9 (2005): 3617–3623. doi: 10.1158/0008-5472.CAN-05-0048.

Ka'ahukane Leite-Ah Yo, K. A., Thomas Hemscheidt, Dana-lynn Ko'omoa Lange, and Alika K. Maunakea. "E hō mai ka 'ike kūpuna no ke ola: Links between Traditional Native Hawaiian Concepts of Health and Epigenetic Research." *Hulili,* under review, 2015.

Kraushaar, D. C., W. Jin, A. Maunakea, B. Abraham, M. Ha, and K. Zhao. "Genome-Wide Incorporation Dynamics Reveal Distinct Categories of Turnover for the Histone Variant H3.3." *Genome Biol* 14, no. 10 (2013), R121. doi: 10.1186/gb-2013-14-10-r121.

Look, Mele A., Mililani K. Trask-Batti, Robert Agres, Marjorie L. Mau, and Joseph Keawe'aimoku Kaholokula. "Health Disparities and Health Care Services." In *Assessment and Priorities for Health and Well-Being in Native Hawaiians and Other Pacific Peoples,* ed. Department of Native Hawaiian Health, pp. 9–19. Honolulu: University of Hawai'i, 2013.

Maunakea, A. K., I. Chepelev, K. Cui, and K. Zhao. "Intragenic DNA Methylation Modulates Alternative Splicing by Recruiting MeCP2 to Promote Exon Recognition." *Cell Research* 23, no. 11 (2013): 1256–1269. doi: 10.1038/cr.2013.110.

Maunakea, A. K., I. Chepelev, and K. Zhao. "Epigenome Mapping in Normal and Disease States." *Circulation Research* 107, no. 3 (2010): 327–339. doi: 10.1161/CIRCRESAHA.110.222463.

Maunakea, A. K., R. P. Nagarajan, M. Bilenky, T. J. Ballinger, C. D'Souza, S. D. Fouse, J. F. Costello, et al. "Conserved Role of Intragenic DNA Methylation in Regulating Alternative Promoters." *Nature* 466, no. 7303 (2010): 253–257. doi: 10.1038/nature09165.

Native Hawaiian Education Council and Ka Haka ʻUla O Keʻelikōlani, College of Hawaiian Language, University of Hawaiʻi at Hilo. "Nā Honua Mauli Ola: Hawaiʻi Guidelines for Culturally Healthy and Responsive Learning Environments." Adopted by the Native Hawaiian Education Council, June 4, 2002.

Pukui, M. K. *ʻŌlelo Noʻeau: Hawaiian Proverbs and Poetical Sayings*. Honolulu: Bishop Museum Press, 1983.

Research, Hula, and Health

Māpuana de Silva, Mele A. Look, Kalehua Tolentino, and Gregory G. Maskarinec

For nearly a decade, biomedical scientists at the University of Hawai'i's John A. Burns School of Medicine's Department of Native Hawaiian Health have been collaborating with kumu hula, cultural practitioners of hula, and communities across Hawai'i to better understand how hula can be the basis for prevention and treatment of heart disease. Research efforts included qualitative studies such as key informant interviews with kumu hula on the relationship of hula with health and well-being[1] and focus groups with cardiac patients post-hospitalization about potential interest in a hula-based rehabilitation program.[2] Other biomedical studies included determining the heart-rate variability of older beginning dancers during a hula class and determination of levels of energy expenditure of different forms of hula.[3] The completion of the initial phase of the Hula Empowering Lifestyle Adaptation (HELA) research study,[4] which evaluated a hula-based cardiac rehabilitation program, was an occasion for wider reflections on lessons learned, directions forward, and, most importantly, ways to preserve cultural integrity when using hula to treat chronic disease. The HELA study was a five-year randomized control trial funded by the prestigious National Institute of Health and utilized the community-based participatory research guidelines to develop and implement study activities. It is the first biomedical investigation to evaluate the cultural practice of hula as part of a health intervention. Kumu hula Māpuana de Silva of Hālau Mōhala 'Ilima[5] has been involved from the conception of these research efforts. To date she has served as research team member, cultural consultant, kumu hula, and advisory committee member on nine different studies of hula and health. Following a performance by her hālau at 'Iolani Palace on July 31, 2012, she shared her thoughts with a department faculty member, Gregory G. Maskarinec, with the assistance of research staff member Kalehua Tolentino. The interview was taped and transcribed. Subsequently, with the assistance of lead investigator and Hālau Mōhala 'Ilima dancer Mele Look, the transcripts were lightly edited into the following reflective narrative.

Can you share your insights on teaching hula as part of a health research study?

Hula is a way of preserving our traditional culture, values, history, everything. The words of our ancestors, all of the songs are written for things that happened or for feelings that people had, things people wished to have happen, there's so much in those *mele.*[6] The words are more important than the movements, but most people don't understand that.

I knew what songs [would] get across to the students better in hula for health classes. For the *'auana* it's "Puamana."[7,8] I didn't even consider another *mele,* mostly because of the words and the story, not because of the choreography or anything else. What we were trying to do was to get folks to enjoy hula and to appreciate Hawaiian culture, and the by-product was better health. The important thing now is we have an example for others to follow. It's such a strong study, anyone who comes along and conducts studies afterward will have to measure up to the HELA project. And so I wanted to choose a song that everyone could identify with, whether they're Hawaiian or not, whether they're born [and] raised here or not, whether they know any of the language or not. "Puamana" was written by Aunty Irmgard [Aluli] for her home. Everyone has a home that is dear to them. It may not be the home you're living in right now, but everyone has a home that they feel is like their home base, so everyone can relate to the song. As we're dancing this song about Aunty's home, the students can relate to the simple imagery about the ocean, the moon, and the love that's shared there. Everybody can identify with all of the things in the song. The poetry is not ambiguous. In the older *mele,* sometimes the words are ambiguous, and are not as literal as "Puamana." There's a lot of Hawaiian vocabulary in "Puamana" that people hear every day or that they hear once in a while and now they know what those words mean. I can teach by using the vocabulary, I can teach by telling the story. Aunty Irmgard passed away less than ten years ago, so older people know who she is. That's another way for them to connect and feel, to identify, with the song. What I was looking for, too, was the old style of music.

With modern hula *'auana* and modern songs, I feel there's a traditional style and then a more contemporary creative style, and I wanted go back to a *mele* that was written in the old style. And then our choreography is really simple. It is one of the simplest choreographies that I have. But what I found, as I was teaching, was that I had to simplify it even more because the important thing was that when the students finished the class, they could actually dance the hula, and that they never felt overwhelmed by the dance or the coordination aspects of it. I would constantly simplify the hula so that the students would get it and they wouldn't feel frustrated by doing a motion on the right and then another motion on the left. Sometimes those of us who dance hula take some things for granted. We don't realize that coordination is really a big stumbling block for many people, and that there are people who have difficulty with hand-eye coordination and reversing motions. It is not a natural thing for everyone. With some groups I could be a little more intricate, and

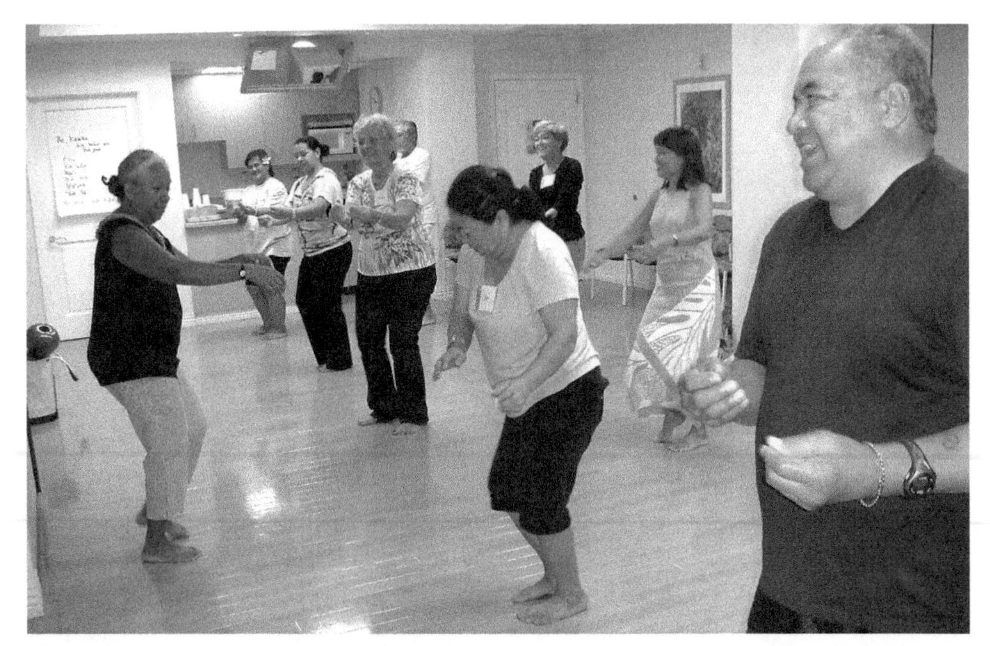

Figure 12.1. Kumu Māpuana de Silva leading hula class for the HELA study at The Queen's Medical Center, 2010. Photo by Fredric Pashkow, used with permission.

with other groups I had to simplify the dance more. Every class was taught a little differently, but that's not really much different than what I do in my hālau.

The stages of learning hula depend on your age, your ability, and your commitment. If you're only going to be in this for a year, then I'm not going to teach you complicated hula. I'm just going to give you a little sprinkling and hope you enjoy it. But in the twelve weeks, it was really important to me that the students in the HELA project could dance "Puamana" at the end because most never danced hula before.[9] Many of them have told me they've danced it with their families, it comes on the radio and they just stand up and dance. They said that because we took the time to write down the choreography, they actually did practice. Because we had hula three times a week, they wanted to come back to the next class and not just have to repeat what they did the class before, so when they copied down the notes, they actually used them. We did "Puamana" first, and then we went into the *kahiko* "Kāwika," which is a little more intense.[10] They would continue to go back to their notes and practice "Puamana" because they didn't want to forget it. And we would use "Puamana" as a warm-up, but I know for a fact that their notes helped, and that's a huge accomplishment. I have students in my hālau who have binders of notes and never look at them [laughs]—but we won't go there.

When my hālau performs, no matter what it's for, we always try to educate.

I always try to bring *mele* that pertain to the situation and think about the purpose of the gathering and what message I want to give; so there's always a message in the *mele* for the dancers as well as the audience. "Kāwika" was the obvious choice because in my hālau, that's the first *kahiko* everyone learns. There are a few exceptions, but for the most part, we try to teach "Kāwika" first. It's our foundation, our base dance. When I was with my kumu, that was a given.[11] Every class that came through learned that *mele*. It is the foundation *mele* of our whole legacy. So it makes sense that I'm trying to give these people more than just choreography. I'm trying to give them a connection to the culture through the line of hula I come from, and that was the perfect way to do it, with "Kāwika."

What was gained through the efforts to use hula to address health conditions?
I want the participants to feel that they have something significant, something special. And I told them, "I'm not here to make you a hula dancer, I'm not here to change your mind about anything, I'm just here to expose you to this. I'm here so you're smarter when you leave than when you walked in." That was really the goal, that they would have more knowledge about hula, and so that they could have a personal experience—they were taught hula, they might never dance hula again, but they can say, "I know because I danced with Kumu Māpuana and I know what it's like." I think it is empowering to these people to have had the experience not just of learning the hula, but learning it with my traditions, my way of thinking, and my way of teaching. Then they can understand about being part of a hula lineage.

When the participants started, most probably couldn't even sing one Hawaiian song from beginning to end. We all sing and have no idea what the words are. For the study, we needed a slow warm-up activity, so I added a sing-walk at the start of every class. I thought that this would be a great opportunity for them to learn a song that everyone sings. We sang all the verses of "Hawai'i Aloha," and I would talk about the words, what they mean, and why this is important to our kūpuna.[12,13] They just said, "Wow! I never knew any of this stuff," and they were so appreciative to be able to sing all the verses.

For Hawaiians this experience can be really empowering, because these are things that a lot of Hawaiians want to know but they don't. Some of them are half Hawaiian, or pure Hawaiian, and they don't feel Hawaiian because they don't know things Hawaiian. For people who live here, it's helping them to understand about the first people of Hawai'i better so that they can better respect the Hawaiian culture. And you know, anyone can dance hula, anyone can speak the language, anyone can sing, and anyone can appreciate all of it. And there's still a different respect that happens to those who descend from the first people who were on this land.

What were benefits, challenges, or risks being involved in a biomedical research study involving hula?

Hula is one of the few activities that can help you with every single aspect of your life. You've got the language, you've got the history, you've got the culture, you've got the movement, you've got the coordination. We know the muscles used in hula are different from other activities, even if you go to the gym, even if you play sports. Hula uses different muscles. And because of the control that you need to dance hula well, or even just to learn a hula, it could definitely help anyone with balance and with breathing. When you get to more intense forms of hula, if you don't choreograph breathing into it, you can lose your breath. That's one of the things I was very conscious about with the HELA project, and I've become more conscious of it in my hālau: choreographing breathing into the exercises that we start with, and choreographing breathing into the dance itself. I've always been conscious of choreographing breathing into the dancing on certain hula, now I'm trying to do it across the board. I've always been conscious of choreographing breathing into my chanting because if I don't, I can't make it to the end of the line, but I've never done it as a regular part of a class. So this study has really made me more aware of so many things.

I've always based my classes on where people are physically. As they get to a higher level, I increase the intensity. What the HELA project made me more conscious of is doing a warm-up, and then a high-intensity period for twenty minutes dancing straight, and then a cool-down for each class. So I have incor-

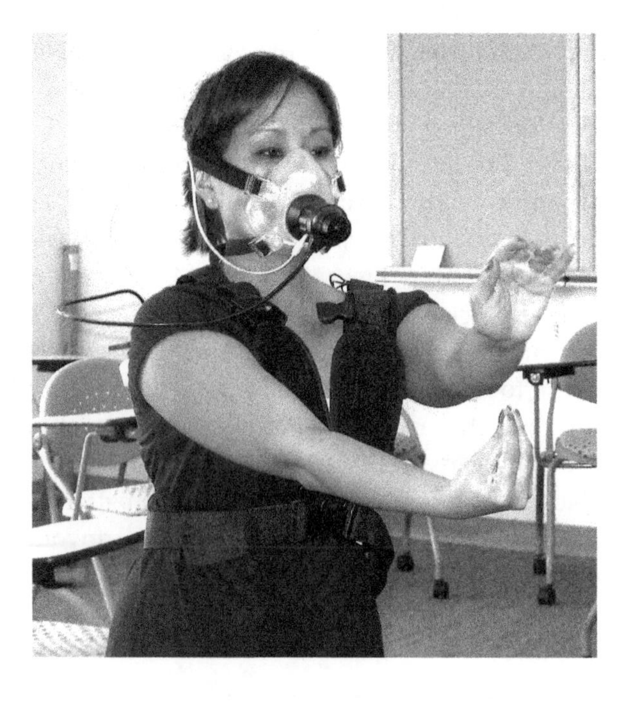

Figure 12.2. Dr. Tricia Marbellos, principal investigator of the MET Study evaluating metabolic measurement equipment, JABSOM, 2011. Photo by Mele Look, used with permission.

porated more of that on a regular basis, especially in the classes for the adults in my hālau who only come to me once a week.

In the HELA project, participants think by coming to hula class it's going to improve their health. You're going to help them to be healthier and to learn how to be healthy and that's why you're there. You're doing it through hula, but hula is just the vehicle. As a kumu, you can't come in to this type of class like you would come in to a hālau class. Perhaps because during the study, we kept saying that we're trying to keep the cultural integrity of a hula class, kumu hula may think they could conduct it like a regular hula class. But there are a lot of differences because you have to make sure all the things are done for the research side, the health side, and also maintain cultural integrity.

There's always been some concern about cultural integrity and traditional hula as opposed to exercise—"hulacize." Hula as a commodity worries me. I'm proud of us as Hawaiians. Hula may be out of control out there in the world, but there are still places where it is really held up high, where it is very respected and it can stand on its own next to a profession like medicine, like research. With so much technology, maintaining the cultural boundaries of hula is nearly impossible, and I'm really sad to say that. I've spent most of my life trying to preserve the traditional cultural aspects of hula.[14] It's how I raised my family. It may be a business, but for me, that's not the first thing it is.

In the HELA project, we are being respected as experts at the same level as the cardiologist. As the cultural expert I am on the same level as these other experts in other fields, and we all come together to work out the plan. I do what I can in the areas that I know, and I try to hold fast to the cultural side of it first and set a good example. One of the things the HELA project did for me was that it made me look at myself as an expert and be okay with that. I still have so much to learn, but I'm sitting at the table with doctors and scientists and they're asking me, "Well, what do you think, Māpuana?" By the time we got to the end of the project, I was really comfortable giving my opinion and making suggestions, and they were really good about not saying, "It has to be like this." They wanted me to lead the changes. It was humbling, but it was a really good place for me to accept where I am at in my career and what I'm doing.

I'm hoping that this study can bring us to the next phase where we can write criteria for what an "expert" in this area is. Just because you teach hula, just because you have traditional knowledge, doesn't mean that you're automatically qualified. You have to go into this kind of project wanting to make a difference. You have to go into it loving those people—whoever walks in the door, you have to love them. You cannot walk in as a kumu; it is clearer to me now that when teaching hula for the HELA project, you walk in with hula credentials that may not be important to the students because these are not hula people. You walk in as the instructor and you have to earn their respect as a kumu, and you have to earn their acknowledgment of you for what you do with them, not what you do outside of class. How are you relating to them? You are their answer to a better life. It is a huge *kuleana*.[15]

What are your thoughts about improving the health of our people, Kānaka Maoli?
I think there are very few health conditions where hula couldn't be a big part of the answer. It's something I've known all these years—this study gives us the evidence. For example, a part of the reason for high blood pressure for us Hawaiians could be that we don't know the people we live with. When I was growing up, I knew everybody in Kailua, so you're not nervous about things around you. You're only nervous if you do something wrong, because somebody's going to see it, your mom's going to find out, and you're going to get a lickin'. But now, you think, "I don't know that person, I don't know if I can trust that person." There's this stress that can develop into hypertension from all the unknowns surrounding you every day. When you bring a community together to address that, I think it helps to deal with hypertension because now there are fewer unknowns. You know people, you see each other on the street, you wave "howzit," and it makes you feel good.

Anything that moves us forward is good. It doesn't have to be perfect, there can be glitches, there can be growing pains, it can evolve as long as we're moving forward and we're making progress. The HELA project lit the fire under all these people and now they're thinking in different ways—how exciting is that? We have to set some minimal standards, and the potential is so great.

Mahalo piha is extended to Fredric Pashkow, MD, Patience Namaka Bacon, Ka'upena Wong, and Kekuni Blaisdell, MD, for their aloha, advice, and guid-

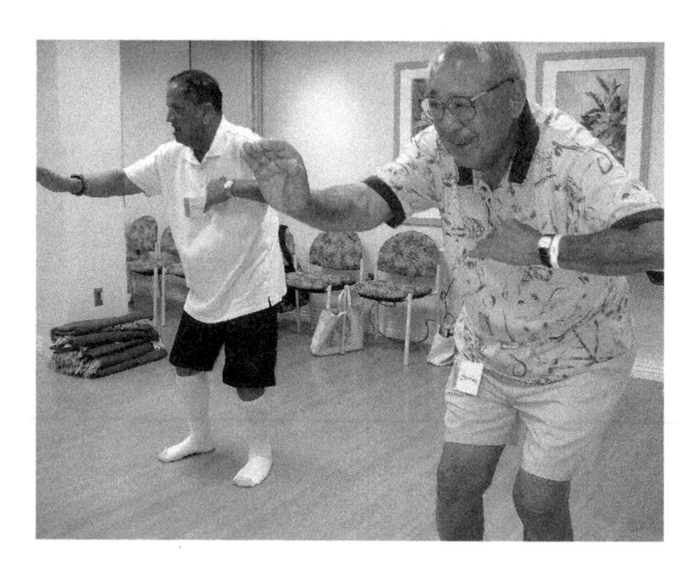

Figure 12.3. Stanley Mah and Daniel Nihipali partipate in the HELA study at The Queen's Medical Center, 2010. Photo by Fredric Pashkow, used with permission.

ance. The authors would also like to acknowledge the funding support of The Queen's Health Systems, the National Institute of Minority Health and Health Disparities (P20MD000173), and the National Lung, Heart, Blood, Institute (R01HL126577). The content is solely the responsibility of the authors and does not necessarily represent the official views of its funders.

NOTES

1. Mele A. Look, Gregory G. Maskarinec, Māpuana de Silva, Todd Seto, Marjorie L. Mau, and Joseph Keawe'aimoku Kaholokula, "Kumu Hula Perspectives on Health," *Hawai'i Journal of Medicine and Public Health* 73, no. 12, Suppl. 3 (2014): 21–25.

2. Mele A. Look, Joseph Keawe'aimoku Kaholokula, Amy Carvalho, Todd Seto, and Māpuana de Silva, "Developing a Culturally Based Cardiac Rehabilitation Program: The HELA Study," *Progress in Community Health Partnerships: Research, Education, and Action* 6, no. 1 (2012): 103–110.

3. Tricia Usagawa, Mele Look, Māpuana de Silva, Christopher Stickley, Joseph Keawe'aimoku Kaholokula, Todd Seto, and Marjorie Mau, "Metabolic Equivalent Determination in the Cultural Dance of Hula," *International Journal of Sports Medicine* 5, no. 35 (2013): 399–402.

4. Gregory G. Maskarinec, Mele A. Look, Kalehua Tolentino, Mililani Trask-Batti, Todd Seto, Māpuana de Silva, and Joseph Keawe'aimoku Kaholokula, "Patient Perspectives on the Hula Empowering Lifestyle Adaptation Study: Benefits of Dancing Hula for Cardiac Rehabilitation," *Health Promotion Practice* 1, no. 1 (2015): 109–114.

5. Hālau Mohala 'Ilima was founded by Māpuana and Kīhei de Silva in 1976 and is located in Ka'ōhao, O'ahu. The hālau has trained thousands of dancers from ages four to eighty years old. It is renowned as a cultural education center with excellence in hula training and traditional language arts and is widely admired for its award-winning dance performances. Also see www.halaumohalailima.com.

6. Mary Kawena Pukui and Samuel H. Elbert, *Hawaiian Dictionary: Hawaiian-English, English-Hawaiian,* rev. and enl. ed. (Honolulu: University of Hawai'i Press, 1986), 245: *mele,* a song, anthem, or chant of any kind; poem, and poetry.

7. Hula is generally categorized into two main forms: 1) *kahiko,* or hula performed to traditional Hawaiian language *oli* (chanting), often accompanied by traditional percussion instruments such as *ipu* or *ipu heke;* and 2) *'auana,* or hula accompanied by singing in English or the Hawaiian language, plus stringed instruments such as guitar, bass, ukulele, piano. Adrienne Kaeppler, *Hula Pahu: Hawaiian Drum Dances* (Honolulu: Bishop Museum Press 1993), 4–33.

8. Irmgard Farden Aluli, an esteemed and prolific songwriter and performer, wrote the iconic Hawaiian song "Puamana" about her childhood home in Lahaina, Maui. It is also the name of her family singing group. Aluli was a longtime resident of Kailua, O'ahu, and a lifelong friend of Māpuana and Kīhei de Silva.

9. The HELA study developed a cardiac rehabilitation program based on beginning halau hula classes and followed the usual prescription for cardiac rehabilitation post-hospitalization of twelve weeks of defined physical activity, three times a week. Look et al., "Developing a Culturally Based Cardiac Rehabilitation Program: The HELA Study."

10. A *mele inoa* or name song for King David Kalākaua is often the first hula *kahiko*

taught to beginning dancers. Some kumu hula purposely select this dance as an initial hula for beginners to acknowledge King Kalākaua's role in revitalizing this cultural practice.

11. Revered kumu hula Maiki Aiu Lake of Hālau Hula o Maiki bestowed the title of kumu hula on Māpuana de Silva in 1975, during the formal *'ūniki* (completion) ceremony of dancers in the hālau's 'Ilima class.

12. The song "Hawai'i Aloha" was written in 1860 by Lorenzo Lyons. It is often the last song sung at Hawaiian gatherings before dispersing. The last line in the chorus states the sentiment of the song: *Mau ke aloha no Hawai'i* (Love for Hawai'i is eternal). Carol Wilcox, Kimo Hussey, Vickey Hollinger, and Puakea Nogelmeier, *He Mele Aloha: A Hawaiian Songbook* (Honolulu: 'Oli'oli Productions, 2003), 45.

13. Pukui and Elbert, *Hawaiian Dictionary,* 186: *kūpuna,* grandparent, ancestor, relative or close friend of the grandparent's generation, grandaunt, or granduncle.

14. Kumu Māpuana de Silva's approach to hula is often noted to be "traditional" in several ways, such as style of dance choreography, focus on language accuracy, skill in language arts, costume selection, and expected behavior of dancers both on and off stage. Also see Jay Hartwell's *Hawaiian People Today: Nā Mamo,* chapter on hula and dance, which describes Hālau Mōhala 'Ilima and Māpuana and Kīhei de Silva's traditional Hawaiian educational focus.

15. Pukui and Elbert, *Hawaiian Dictionary,* 179: *kuleana,* privilege, concern, right, or responsibility.

BIBLIOGRAPHY

Hartwell, Jay. *Nā Mamo: Hawaiian People Today.* Honolulu: 'Ai Pōhaku Press, 1996.

Kaeppler, Adrienne L. *Hula Pahu: Hawaiian Drum Dances.* Honolulu: Bishop Museum Press, 1993.

Look, Mele A., Joseph Keawe'aimoku Kaholokula, Amy Carvalho, Todd Seto, and Māpuana de Silva. "Developing a Culturally Based Cardiac Rehabilitation Program: The HELA Study." *Progress in Community Health Partnerships: Research, Education, and Action* 6, no. 1 (2012): 103–110.

Look, Mele A., Gregory G. Maskarinec, Māpuana de Silva, Todd Seto, Marjorie L. Mau, and Joseph Keawe'aimoku Kaholokula. "Kumu Hula Perspectives on Health." *Hawai'i Journal of Medicine and Public Health* 73, no. 12, Suppl. 3 (2014): 21–25.

Maskarinec, Gregory G., Mele A. Look, Kalehua Tolentino, Mililani Trask-Batti, Todd Seto, Māpuana de Silva, and Joseph Keawe'aimoku Kaholokula. "Patient Perspectives on the Hula Empowering Lifestyle Adaptation Study: Benefits of Dancing Hula for Cardiac Rehabilitation." *Health Promotion Practice* 16, no. 1 (2015): 109–114.

Pukui, Mary Kawena, and Samuel H. Elbert. *Hawaiian Dictionary: Hawaiian-English, English-Hawaiian,* rev. and enl. ed. Honolulu: University of Hawai'i Press, 1986.

Usagawa, Tricia, Mele Look, Māpuana de Silva, Christopher Stickley, Joseph Keawe'aimoku Kaholokula, Todd Seto, and Marjorie Mau. "Metabolic Equivalent Determination in the Cultural Dance of Hula." *International Journal of Sports Medicine* 5, no. 35 (2013): 399–402.

Wilcox, Carol, Kimo Hussey, Vicky Hollinger, and Puakea Nogelmeier. *He Mele Aloha: A Hawaiian Songbook.* Honolulu: 'Oli'Oli Productions, 2003.

Contributors

Note: the University of Hawai'i at Mānoa John A. Burns School of Medicine is noted below as JABSOM, and the University of Hawai'i at Mānoa as UHM.

Nina Leialoha Beckwith, MEd, is a kama'āina from windward O'ahu. She graduated from Kalāheo High School in 2005 and received a bachelor of science degree in neurobiology, physiology, and behavior from the University of California, Davis in 2010. Subsequently, she served as a seventh-grade science teacher at Wai'anae Intermediate School, while earning her master of education degree from UHM. With a deep passion for improving the wellness of Native Hawaiian communities, she started working with Drs. Reni Soon and Jennifer Elia in the Department of Obstetrics, Gynecology, and Women's Health on a Native Hawaiian family planning research study, and in 2015 she completed her first year of medical school at JABSOM. Her goals are to serve in rural areas throughout Hawai'i and to incorporate traditional forms of healing into her future medical practice. She loves hula and is a member of Hālau Nā Pualei O Likolehua.

Richard Kekuni Blaisdell, MD, was professor emeritus of the Department of Medicine and consultant to the Department of Native Hawaiian Health at JABSOM. He graduated from Kamehameha Schools for Boys in 1942 and earned a bachelor's degree in pre-medicine at the University of Redlands and graduated from the University of Chicago Medical School in 1948. He was a medical officer in the Korean War in Japan and Taiwan from 1957 to 1959 and a hematology researcher at the Atomic Bomb Casualty Commission in Hiroshima and Nagasaki, where he conducted studies on the late effects of radiation. After an internship at Johns Hopkins Medical School, a medical residency at Tulane University, and a pathology residency at Duke University Medical Center, he returned to the University of Chicago Medical School as an assistant professor of medicine. He was recruited back to Hawai'i to become the first chair of the Department of Medicine at the newly established University of Hawai'i School of Medicine. While in this position, he helped to establish clinical training programs in Saipan, Palau, Chuuk, Pohnpei, Guam, and Okinawa. In 1983, Kekuni authored the influential *E Ola Mau* report on the declining health of Kānaka Maoli and participated in drafting the Native Hawaiian

Healthcare Act, enacted by Congress in 1988. He is co-founder of E Ola Mau, a Native Hawaiian health provider association and a charter member of 'Ahahui o nā Kauka, an association of Native Hawaiian physicians. He served on the boards of trustees for two Native Hawaiian health-care systems and participated in the development of JABSOM's Department of Native Hawaiian Health. He has received numerous awards including the Ka'ōnohi award from Papa Ola Lōkahi, the Alumni Service Award from the University of Chicago, the Lifetime Achievement Award from the Asian and Pacific Islander American Health Forum, the Living Treasure of Hawai'i designation from Honpa Hongwanji Mission of Hawai'i, the Physician of the Year award from the Hawai'i Medical Association, the 'Ō'ō Award from the Native Hawaiian Chamber of Commerce, the David Malo award from the West Honolulu Rotary Club, and the I Ulu Ke Kumu award from the Hawai'inuiākea School of Hawaiian Knowledge at UHM.

Kalani Brady, MPH, MD, is a Native Hawaiian physician, television news correspondent, musician, and actor. A graduate of St. Louis High School, Dr. Brady earned a bachelor's degree from Harvard University in engineering and applied physics, a master of public health degree in biostatistics epidemiology from UHM, and a medical doctor degree from the University of Pennsylvania. He is currently an associate professor in the Department of Native Hawaiian Health at JABSOM and is cohost of the "Ask the Doctor" weekly segment on broadcast television news. Dr. Brady is chief of medical staff at the Kalaupapa clinic on Moloka'i, which serves all residents of Kalaupapa. He also continues to see patients in his practice at the Lau Ola Clinic in downtown Honolulu. Dr. Brady is a fellow of the American College of Physicians and is board certified in internal medicine.

Dee-Ann Carpenter, MD, is a Native Hawaiian physician specializing in internal medicine. She received her bachelor's degree from UHM and completed the 'Imi Ho'ōla Program to graduate with an MD from JABSOM. Dr. Carpenter did her residency with the UH Integrated Medical Residency Program and was one of two fourth-year residents in the inaugural year of the Senior Residency in Ambulatory Care Program. She currently practices internal medicine at the Lau Ola Clinic and is an assistant professor in the Department of Native Hawaiian Health at JABSOM. She enjoys teaching clinical medicine and is part of the C3 Team that teaches the cultural competency curriculum. She is a board member of the 'Ahahui o nā Kauka and the founding president and current board member of the Friends of 'Imi Ho'ōla. Dr. Carpenter was recently awarded the MESRE Award for Excellence for outstanding oral presentation of an educational innovation in medical education at the 2014 WGEA conference. She is the proud mother of two beautiful children, Marin and Pono.

Rebecca Delafield, MPH, is a clinical research coordinator with the Department of Native Hawaiian Health. Born in the Northern Mariana Islands and raised in the Midwestern United States, Rebecca moved to Hawai'i shortly after graduating with her master in public health from the University of North Carolina at Chapel Hill. She started working with the Department of Native Hawaiian Health (DNHH) in 2008 and is currently coordinating efforts to disseminate the evidence-based interventions developed and tested by the PILI 'Ohana Partnership to more islands and communities throughout Hawai'i. Rebecca's work has focused on community-based research studies dealing with health disparities, specifically those of rural Native Hawaiian and Pacific Islander populations. Prior to coming to DNHH, she worked in community health clinics and with larger health organizations coordinating statewide programmatic initiatives. Her work in Hawai'i has consistently involved collaboration with a multitude of community-based agencies serving Native Hawaiians and Pacific Islanders.

Māpuana de Silva founded the esteemed Hālau Mōhala 'Ilima in 1976. Located in Ka'ōhao, O'ahu, the hālau has trained thousands of dancers from ages four to eighty-plus. It is renowned as a cultural education center with excellence in hula training and traditional language arts and is widely admired for its award-winning dance performances. Kumu hula Māpuana was trained by revered kumu hula Maiki Aiu Lake of Hālau Hula o Maiki and was bestowed the title and privileges of kumu hula in 1975 during the formal 'ūniki completion ceremony of the hālau's 'Ilima class. Kumu hula Māpuana has collaborated with JABSOM on hula and health research studies since 2007. She has served as a research team member, cultural consultant, kumu hula, and advisory committee member on nine different hula and health studies. In 2014, she and husband Kīhei were recognized by the Hawai'inuiākea School of Hawaiian Knowledge at UHM with the I Ulu I Ke Kumu award for outstanding contributions to Hawaiian education and well-being.

Sasha Naomi Kehaulani Hayashi Treschuk Fernandes, MD, was born and raised on O'ahu and has strong ties to Hilo where her grandparents lived. Her son, Gabriel, inspires her to follow the path of her parents, Ed and Lori Treschuk, who work for human rights, peace, and Hawaiian land rights. After obtaining her bachelor of arts degree in sociology at Brandeis University, she attended JABSOM and trained at Kapi'olani Medical Center and Kōkua Kalihi Valley community health clinic to become a pediatric physician. In 2010, Dr. Fernandes joined the Native Hawaiian Center of Excellence (NHCOE) as lead faculty for the Native Hawaiian Student Pathway to Medicine program and became one of the leaders of the Native Hawaiian Interdisciplinary Health program. Dr. Fernandes loves working with her NHCOE 'ohana to empower haumāna of all ages to pursue their calling to uplift our communities by restoring wellness in our beloved Hawai'i.

Courtney Kielemaikalani Gaddis, MSIII, was born and raised in Honolulu. She is currently a third-year medical student at JABSOM. She graduated from Kalani High School in 2007 and earned her bachelor's degree in biology from UHM, where she was a student athlete playing for the Rainbow Wahine basketball team. She began dancing hula at the age of four with Hālau Hula O Maiki, and continues to share her love for hula through dancing.

Akolea K. Ioane, MD, was born and raised on Hawai'i Island and was among the first group of Native Hawaiian children beyond the island of Ni'ihau to be educated entirely in Hawaiian from kindergarten through high school since the 1800s. She is part of the second graduating class of Ke Kula 'O Nawahīokalani'ōpu'u Hawaiian immersion school. Having been raised in both Hawaiian and English, she is a native speaker of Hawaiian. She is currently a second-year family medicine resident at the VCU-Shenandoah family practice residency. She earned her bachelor's degree in nursing at UH Hilo and completed her MD at JABSOM. She is a mother of two and, prior to becoming a physician, had dedicated her life to perpetuating Hawaiian language and culture. Her contribution to this piece is a reflection on bridging those two worlds.

'Ānela K. Nacapoy Iwane is from He'eia, O'ahu. She is a wife, mother, daughter, sister, aunty, hula dancer, and kumu kaiāpuni at Ke Kula Kaiapuni o Hau'ula. She graduated from UHM and is dedicated to the perpetuation of the Hawaiian language and culture, especially in Native Hawaiian education. She is an active participant in the 'Aha Kauleo.

Marcus Kawika Iwane, MD, is from Mililani (Waipi'o), O'ahu. He graduated from JABSOM in 2010. He completed his internal medicine training at UHM's Internal Medicine Residency Program and served as a chief medical resident at the Kuakini Medical Center. He is a physician practicing at the Kaiser Nānāikeola Clinic in Nānākuli and serves on the board for Ka 'Ahahui o nā Kauka. He and his 'ohana currently reside in Pu'uloa. Together with his wife, 'Ānela, he composed the oli "Ki'eki'e Lanihuli" for the very first 'Aha Ho'omolo Kīhei ceremony at his graduation, now an annual tradition at JABSOM commencement exercises.

Puni Jackson and her family are the caretakers at Ho'oulu 'Āina, Kōkua Kalihi Valley's 100-acre nature preserve where health programming includes mālama 'āina education, indigenous food and plant production, removal and repurposing of invasive plant species, the cultivation of Hawaiian medicinal herbs, and ancient site restoration. A widely exhibited artist, Puni has shown her work locally and internationally over the past ten years. Pervading themes in her work are her ancestry and heritage as an indigenous woman of Hawai'i, aloha, and the relationship between 'āina and kanaka.

Puni says, "the valley where I was born is Nu'uanu, my 'āina is Pu'unui, my rain is Pōpōkapa, my wind is Kūla'ikanaka. I came to this realm he wahine, he Hawai'i. My home has moved two valleys, four-and-a-half miles. I have become a mother, a wife, a farmer, a forester, a chanter, an agrophilosopher, a painter, a carver, an advocate, a healer, an organizer, a fighter, and a lover. My wind is Haupe'epe'e, my rain is Ko'ilipilipi, my 'āina is Māluawai, the valley where I live, where my children were born, is Kalihilihi o Laumiha."

Nanette Kapulani Mossman Judd, PhD, MPH, RN, is a professor emeritus of the Department of Native Hawaiian Health at JABSOM. She has served Hawai'i's health community for over thirty-five years. As former director of 'Imi Ho'ōla Post-Baccalaureate Program, she assisted disadvantaged graduate students pursue their dreams of becoming a physician and as such, Dr. Judd has mentored, shaped, and supported over 250 Native Hawaiian and Pacific Islander students, making 'Imi Ho'ōla a model program across the United States and throughout the Pacific. Many of those students are leaders today and serve as kumu to a new generation of young physicians. She is the recipient of several awards, including the Regional Health Administrator's Special Service Award under the U.S. Department of Health and Human Services, and was recently recognized by the Hawai'inuiākea School of Hawaiian Knowledge at UHM with the I Ulu I Ke Kumu award. Her visionary legacy is one of building diversity while increasing the number of physicians in Hawai'i's most rural and underserved areas.

Joseph Keawe'aimoku Kaholokula, PhD, is the eldest son of Lawrence Pauahi Kaholokula and Beverly Leilani Lyons. He is a cultural practitioner with Hale Mua o Kūali'i, a professor and the chair of Native Hawaiian Health at JABSOM, a behavioral scientist, a health equity advocate, and a licensed clinical psychologist. He received his doctoral degree in clinical psychology from UHM in 2003 and completed a clinical health psychology postdoctoral fellowship in 2004 at the Tripler Army Medical Center. Using community-based participatory research (CBPR) approaches, he works closely with Native Hawaiian and Pacific Islander communities to develop culturally relevant and community-led health promotion strategies to reduce the risk for diabetes and heart disease. He also studies the effects of discrimination and other socio-cultural stressors on the health and well-being of Native Hawaiians. As a member of several community boards and committees, he is a strong advocate for improving the social and cultural determinants of health for Native Hawaiians.

Martina Leialoha Kamaka, MD, is a Native Hawaiian family physician. She is a graduate of the Kamehameha Schools, the University of Notre Dame (BA), and JABSOM (MD). She is board certified in family medicine and completed her residency training in Lancaster, Pennsylvania. She was in private practice both in Pennsylvania and, later, back home in Hawai'i. She is currently an associate professor in the Department of Native Hawaiian Health at JABSOM pursuing her interest in cultural competency training and indigenous health that she has been working on since 1999. She is the director for the DNHH Cultural Competency Curriculum Development project that focuses on cultural competency training for medical students and residents. She is a founding member and president of the 'Ahahui o nā Kauka and serves on the international steering committee for the Pacific Region Indigenous Doctors Congress.

Leimomi Noel Kanagusuku, MSII, was born and raised in Wai'anae, O'ahu. She attended Kamehameha Schools Kapālama and graduated from Stanford University with a bachelor's degree in human biology with a focus on health in underserved communities. She is a recent graduate of the 'Imi Ho'ōla Program and is currently a second-year medical student at JABSOM. She aspires to practice primary care in her hometown, promote public health measures, and encourage Native Hawaiian youth to pursue higher education in hopes of improving overall health measures for the people of Hawai'i.

C. Malina Kaulukukui, MSW, is a faculty member at the Myron B. Thompson School of Social Work at UHM, where she coordinates the Hawaiian Learning Program, a workforce development initiative that provides enhanced cultural training to Native Hawaiian MSW students. She is also a member of JABSOM's Cultural Competency Curriculum Development project, where she assists in the development and implementation of cultural competency initiatives such as the cultural immersion program for first-year medical students. Ms. Kaulukukui is a cultural practitioner of *lua* and a kumu hula, teaching in the Kaka'ako area. Under the tutelage of Richard and Lynette Paglinawan, recognized *ho'oponopono* practitioners, she is completing advanced mentoring in *ho'oponopono*. She has developed curricula for holistically oriented treatment with substance-abusing women at the Salvation Army Family Treatment Services utilizing Hawaiian cultural values and practices as the foundation for these interventions. She continues to use her knowledge and skills in developing curricula that integrate Hawaiian practices with Western perspectives.

Dana-Lynn Ko'omoa, PhD, is a Native Hawaiian biomedical researcher. She graduated from McKinley High School, completed her BSc degree at San Diego

State University in cellular and molecular biology, and earned her doctorate at Brown University in molecular pharmacology, physiology, and biotechnology. Dr. Ko'omoa completed her postdoctoral training at the UH Cancer Center and at the Abramson's Research Center at the University of Pennsylvania. She is currently an assistant professor at the Daniel K. Inouye College of Pharmacy at UH Hilo. Her research involves elucidating the mechanisms that promote the progression of cancer and identifying novel targets for the development of more effective chemotherapeutic agents and treatment strategies for advanced stage, high-risk, and drug-resistant cancers. Dr. Ko'omoa also participates in the Uluākea and Ho'okahua programs at UH Hilo to increase diversity in STEM fields, gain a more authentic and practical understanding of indigenous ways of learning, and transform UH Hilo into a Hawaiian place of learning.

Malia-Susanne Lee, MD, graduated from UHM, where she received her bachelor's degree in biology. She is a former 'Imi Ho'ōla Post-Baccalaureate Program student and Native Hawaiian Health Scholar. She received her medical doctor degree from JABSOM, then completed her residency at the Loma Linda University Medical Center and the University of Hawai'i Family Practice Residencies. She committed fifteen years of service as a family medicine provider in community health and completed a fellowship in education and research with the Native Hawaiian Center of Excellence and the Office of Medical Education, where she focused on adolescent education and its impact on health and the community. She has been the director of the Native Hawaiian Center of Excellence since February 2015. She is a singer/songwriter and a Nā Hōkū Hanohano award nominee for her first album, *Eyes of a Stranger,* which was inspired by her patients and family.

Winona Kaalouahi Mesiona Lee, MD, has served as director of the medical education division of the Department of Native Hawaiian Health at JABSOM since 2011. Dr. Lee oversees two key diversity programs, the 'Imi Ho'ōla Post-Baccalaureate Program and the Native Hawaiian Center of Excellence, both of which promote the success of underrepresented and disadvantaged students in medicine and other health professions. Dr. Lee was born and raised in 'Ewa Beach and is a proud graduate of Kamehameha Schools Kapālama campus. She earned her bachelor's degree in biology and her MD at UHM. Dr. Lee is a board-certified pediatrician, and prior to joining the Department of Native Hawaiian Health provided primary care services to children in foster care. Dr. Lee's primary interests include health-care workforce diversity, medical professionalism, mentorship of at-risk youth, and cultural competency.

Mele A. Look, MBA, has worked as a health researcher, community advocate, and health administrator for Native Hawaiian and Pacific Islander communities for over thirty-five years and has been a cultural practitioner of hula for more than forty-five years. As director for community engagement at the Center for Native and Pacific Health Disparities Research (P20) and the Department of Native Hawaiian Health at JABSOM, Ms. Look founded and facilitates the Ulu Network, a cardiometabolic health community coalition which has grown to thirty community-based organizations serving Native Hawaiians and Pacific Islanders at over seventy sites across Hawai'i and the continental United States. Ms. Look earned an undergraduate degree in American studies from UHM and a master's degree in business administration from the University of California at Berkeley. Ms. Look has received training for hula, cultural protocol, and language arts at Hālau Mōhala 'Ilima for nearly twenty years. In a formal hula graduation ceremony, the *'uniki 'ailolo,* Ms. Look was recently awarded the title of *'olapa* (accomplished dancer).

Gregory G. Maskarinec, PhD, is a cultural anthropologist who teaches in the Department of Native Hawaiian Health and the Department of Family Medicine and Community Health at JABSOM. He has conducted research on traditional medicine, medical education, and contemporary medical systems in Nepal, Bangladesh, Kyrgyzstan, Palau, American Samoa, the Federated States of Micronesia (Yap, Chuuk, Pohnpei, and Kosrae), and the Republic of the Marshall Islands, as well as in Hawai'i and Arkansas. The author of several books and many articles, his work on Nepal was honored with an award from the late king of Nepal, Birendra Bir Bikram Shah Dev, on the recommendation of the Nepal Royal Academy. His work also gained him an honorary degree of Sanskritic scholarship by the late Yogi Naraharinath. He is an affiliate scholar of the Centre National de la Recherche Scientific in Paris and has taught as a visiting professor at the following institutions: Tribhuvan University in Kathmandu, Nepal; Asian University for Women in Chittagong, Bangladesh; University of Paris X in Nanterre; and the University of Zürich in Switzerland.

Alika K. Maunakea, PhD, is a Native Hawaiian biomedical researcher who has conducted epigenetic research in mammalian systems for over fifteen years, during which he has made several important contributions that have helped advance the field of epigenetics, in particular the development and application of novel high-throughput, genome-wide technologies that survey DNA methylation and histone modifications, both central components of epigenetic processes, and discovery of novel roles for DNA methylation in regulating alternative promoter usage, and in pre-mRNA splicing. Currently Dr. Maunakea is applying epigenomic information toward understanding the mechanistic relationships of gene-environment interactions that underlie the development of disease. Dr. Maunakea plays a leading role in understanding how the environment interacts with epigenetic processes that may underlie diseases of health disparities, including diabetes and cardiovascular disease, with the hope that these translational research efforts will contribute to the development of more effective targeted diagnostic, preventative, and therapeutic strategies to improve the health of underserved communities. His interest in health science was due in part to his upbringing in Native Hawaiian culture, values, and traditional practices of medicine taught to him by his great-grandmother Katherine Maunakea in Nānākuli, O'ahu. After graduating from Kamehameha Schools, where he discovered an anti-cancer compound in a Hawaiian medicinal plant, Dr. Maunakea went on to receive his BSc degree in biology at Creighton University and doctorate in biomedical sciences at the University of California, San Francisco. He completed postdoctoral training at the National Institutes of Health in 2012 and has since joined JABSOM and Hawai'inuiākea School of Hawaiian Knowledge at UHM as an assistant professor in the Department of Native Hawaiian Health conducting epigenomic research and training the next generation of underrepresented minority students in health sciences.

Diane S. L. Paloma, MBA, PhD, is the director of the Native Hawaiian Health Program at The Queen's Health Systems, a hospital system that includes three rural hospitals and Hawai'i's only tertiary care center. Since 2006, her responsibilities have included managing clinical initiatives, health-care training, health disparities' translational research, and community outreach to Hawai'i's diverse Native Hawaiian population. A Kamehameha Schools graduate, she received her bachelor's degree in physiological science, a master's degree in business with an emphasis in management, and a doctorate in health-care administration. Diane has been in the health field since 1995 and has consistently combined her passion for Native Hawaiian culture with the health and medical fields. Her experience in health care includes administration in a clinical practice, management in health insurance, and service as a faculty member at JABSOM's Department of Native Hawaiian Health.

Karen K. Sakamoto, MS, has been an educator, student advocate, and consultant in the area of student learning and development for over thirty-five years at UHM. She earned a bachelor's degree in education from UHM with a focus on special education and a master's degree in pupil personnel services from California State University at Long Beach. She currently serves as the learning specialist for both the 'Imi Ho'ōla Program and the Office of Student Affairs at JABSOM. Her responsibilities include fostering effective learning and critical thinking skills, administering and analyzing learning and personal awareness assessments, and creating individualized education plans. She has been instrumental in creating and implementing student development services such as mentoring at JABSOM. Her prior experience includes serving as coordinator of the Learning Assistance Center in the Office of Student Affairs at UHM and serving as a resource and consultant to campus programs, academic departments, and community organizations.

Shelley Soong, MEd, MPH, was born and raised on the island of O'ahu. She earned a master of public health degree in health promotion from San Diego State University and a master of education degree from UHM. She has worked on various health intervention programs through JABSOM's Department of Tropical Medicine and Department of Native Hawaiian Health, and through San Diego State University's Institute for Behavioral and Community Health and Center for Behavioral and Community Health. She is a licensed teacher, and prior to working in the Department of Native Hawaiian Health she worked as a middle and high school teacher in the Hawai'i State Department of Education. Her areas of interest include health and cultural promotion among Native Hawaiians and creating and implementing education and research training programs for Native Hawaiians to increase the number of Native Hawaiians in the health workforce.

Patrice Ming-Lei Tim Sing, MD, was born and raised in Hilo, Hawai'i. She is a graduate of Kamehameha Schools, having boarded at the Kapālama campus. She earned her bachelor of science degree in biology at the University of the Pacific. Dr. Tim Sing is a graduate of JABSOM and is currently an assistant professor with the 'Imi Ho'ōla Program. She is also a practicing internist and pediatrician for Kaiser Permanente Medical Group and functions as their lead MD for diversity and inclusion.

Kalehua Tolentino comes from the verdant lands nestled between the Wai'anae and Ko'olau mountain ranges amidst landscapes of red dirt, sugarcane, and pineapple fields. Low-lying clouds and misty rains welcome her in the morning, and orange-colored sunsets and starry nights bid her *a hui hou* at the end of the day. She has laughed, lived, and loved beside peers and patients at The Queen's Medical Center for over thirty years. Currently, she is a coordinator focusing on the medical center's staff development and is pursuing a degree in instructional design with a goal to create online learning that engages and provides information and skills for staff. Kalehua has danced hula for over twenty years with nā kumu hula Mae Ulalia Loebenstein and Maelia Loebenstein Carter at Ka Pā Hula O Kauanoe O Wa'ahila. She participated in the HELA study and the Ola Hou i Ka Hula: Hypertension and Hula Project as part of her academic training. She seeks to establish bridges between medicine and culture to improve the health and well-being of the people of Hawai'i and across the world.

Claire Townsend Ing, DrPH, is an assistant professor at the Department of Native Hawaiian Health at UH-JABSCOM. She has long held academic and research interests in health disparities informed by a social determinants framework. She was awarded a bachelor's degree in anthropology from Pomona College, an MPH in health behavior and health education from the University of North Carolina at Chapel Hill, and a DrPH in community-based and translational research from UHM. For the past seven years, Dr. Townsend Ing has coordinated several community-based participatory research (CBPR) projects at the Department of Native Hawaiian Health. Notable among these is the NIH-funded Partnerships to Improve Lifestyle Interventions (PILI) 'Ohana Project, a NIMHD-funded, CBPR initiative by the PILI 'Ohana Partnership (POP) to address obesity and related disparities in Native Hawaiians and other Pacific Islanders. The POP developed and tested two culturally congruent, community-placed, evidence-based health promotion programs and is currently working to disseminate these interventions to community-based organizations across the State. Additionally, Dr. Townsend Ing is working to build her research in the field of health disparities and has had several successfully funded pilot CBPR projects. These projects included a test of the effectiveness of a semi-structured social support group in maintaining or improving diabetes management, a homestead health survey, and an adaptation of the PILI 'Ohana healthy lifestyle intervention for web-based delivery.

Kelli-Ann Frank Voloch, MD, was born and raised in Makakilo, O'ahu, and is a graduate of the Kamehameha Schools Kapālama campus. She earned a bachelor of science degree in biology and psychology from the College of Notre Dame and became a graduate of the 'Imi Ho'ōla Post-Baccalaureate Program, receiving her medical doctor degree from JABSOM. She has served as an assistant professor in the Department of Native Hawaiian Health for the 'Imi Ho'ōla Program since 2005 and as a pediatrician at the Wai'anae Coast Comprehensive Health Center since 2000. She is involved in many Westside community projects as a mentor and advocate to improve the health and educational status of Hawai'i's keiki and loves to inspire young children and adolescents to believe in their dreams.

Kamuela Werner, MPH, is a research assistant in the Community Engagement Division of JABSOM's Department of Native Hawaiian Health. He develops, implements, and disseminates scientific and medical information to allied health professionals within the Ulu Network, a community coalition of thirty health organizations with over seventy sites that serve Native Hawaiians and other Pacific Islanders in Hawai'i and on the continental United States. He also serves as po'o in the department's stewardship activities related to the medical school's *māla lā'au lapa'au,* a medicinal plant garden used as a living outdoor classroom that provides opportunities for learners to appreciate Hawaiian ancestral knowledge and reconnection to the land. He has academic and professional experience in natural resource management with a focus on native plant conservation and recently completed a master's degree in public health specializing in Native Hawaiian and indigenous populations at UHM. He is from the Wai'anae Coast and now resides in Waimānalo, O'ahu.

Vanessa S. Wong, MD, is an assistant professor in the Department of Native Hawaiian Health and the Office of Medical Education at JABSOM. She is a graduate of the 'Imi Ho'ōla Program and the UH Family Medicine Residency Training Program. As a family physician, she is committed to improving the health of families and communities, particularly those with significant health disparities. She has worked closely with the U.S. Affiliated Pacific Islands in helping communities develop and implement comprehensive cancer control plans and serves as a clinical preceptor for the JABSOM medical student–run homeless clinics. Her current area of interest is medical student education with an emphasis on cultural competency and health disparities.

Benjamin Young, MD, graduated from Roosevelt High School in Honolulu. He earned his bachelor of arts degree in English literature from Milligan College in Tennessee and his medical doctor degree from Howard University in Washington, DC. He trained at JABSOM's medical residency program and became the very first Native Hawaiian psychiatrist. His professional positions at JABSOM include dean of students and executive director of the Native Hawaiian Center of Excellence. Other professional positions include vice-president for student affairs for the University of Hawai'i System, chief of medical staff for Castle Medical Center, president of the Polynesian Voyaging Society, and president of the National Council for Diversity in the Health Professions. In 1972, Dr. Young created the revolutionary 'Imi Ho'ōla Program at JABSOM to increase the numbers of Native Hawaiians and Pacific Islanders in medicine. As part of his Polynesian Voyaging Society leadership, he helped create and build the renowned voyaging canoe *Hōkūle'a* and was the crew physician on its first voyage in 1976. He has received numerous awards including the Distinguished Historian award from the Hawaiian Historical Society, the Living Treasure of Hawai'i designation from the Honpa Hongwanji Mission of Hawai'i, the Ka'ōnohi award from Papa Ola Lōkahi, the 'Ō'ō award from the Native Hawaiian Chamber of Commerce, the David Malo award from the West Honolulu Rotary Club, and the I Ulu I Ke Kumu award from the Hawai'inuiākea School of Hawaiian Knowledge at UHM.

Hawai'inuiākea Series

The Hawai'inuiākea Series provides a multidisciplinary venue for the work of scholars and practitioners from the Hawaiian community, a platform for thinkers and doers who grapple with real-world queries, challenges, and strategies. Each volume features articles on a thematic topic from diverse fields such as economics, education, family resources, government, health, history, land and natural resources, psychology, religion, and sociology. Each volume includes kupuna reflections, current viewpoints, and original creative expression.

No. 1 *I Ulu I Ke Kumu*, Puakea Nogelmeier, editor, 2011.
No. 2 *I Ulu I Ka 'Āina*, Jonathan Osorio, editor, 2013.
No. 3 *'Ike Ulana Lau Hala*, Lia O'Neill M. A. Keawe, Marsha MacDowell, and C. Kurt Dewhurst, editors, 2014.
No. 4 *Kanaka 'Oiwi Methodologies*, Katrina-Ann R. Kapā'anaokalāokeola Nākoa Oliveira and Erin Kahunawaika'ala Wright, editors, 2016.

Proposals for volume themes may be submitted to:
Hawai'inuiākea School of Hawaiian Knowledge
Hawai'inuiākea Series
Office of the Dean
2450 Maile Way
Spalding 454
Honolulu, Hawaii 96822

http://manoa.hawaii.edu/hshk/